MAINTAINING EFFECTIVE
TOKEN ECONOMIES

Some of the material in this book was presented at a symposium at the annual convention of the Association for the Advancement of Behavior Therapy in New York City.

MAINTAINING
EFFECTIVE
TOKEN ECONOMIES

Edited by

ROGER L. PATTERSON, Ph.D.

Associate Professor
Research and Evaluation Section
Florida Mental Health Institute
Tampa, Florida

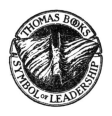

CHARLES C THOMAS · PUBLISHER
Springfield · Illinois · U.S.A.

RC
489
. B4
M34

Published and Distributed Throughout the World by
CHARLES C THOMAS • PUBLISHER
Bannerstone House
301-327 East Lawrence Avenue, Springfield, Illinois, U.S.A.

© *1976, by* CHARLES C THOMAS • PUBLISHER
ISBN 0-398-03435-4
Library of Congress Catalog Card Number: 75-8624

B4 T

With THOMAS BOOKS *careful attention is given to all details of
manufacturing and design. It is the Publisher's desire to present books
that are satisfactory as to their physical qualities and artistic possibilities
and appropriate for their particular use.* THOMAS BOOKS *will be true
to those laws of quality that assure a good name and good will.*

Printed in the United States of America
W-11

Library of Congress Cataloging in Publication Data
Main entry under title:

Maintaining effective token economies.

Based on papers presented at a symposium at the annual
convention of the Association for the Advancement of
Behavior Therapy in New York City in Oct. 1972.
    Bibliography: p.
    Includes index.
    1. Behavior therapy—Congresses. 2.   Reinforcement
(Psychology)—Congresses.   I.   Patterson, Roger L.
II.   Association for Advancement of Behavior Therapy.
RC489-B4M34   616.8'914   75-8624
ISBN 0-398-03435-4

To Bob Liberman, whose idea started this

CONTRIBUTORS

JOHN M. ATTHOWE, JR., Ph.D.: Rutgers Medical School, New Brunswick, New Jersey.

VAL BAKER: Camarillo Neuropsychiatric Institute Research Program, Camarillo, California.

JOHN R. DAVIS: Camarillo Neuropsychiatric Institute Research Program, Camarillo, California.

JOHN P. FOREYT, Ph.D.: Florida State Hospital, Chatahoochee, Florida; and Florida State University, Tallahassee, Florida.

ALAN E. KAZDIN, Ph.D.: Pennsylvania State University, University Park, Pennsylvania.

TITUS McINNIS, Ph.D.: University of Illinois, Urbana, Illinois.

ROGER L. PATTERSON, Ph.D.: Florida Mental Health Institute, Tampa, Florida.

CHARLES J. WALLACE, Ph.D.: Camarillo Neuropsychiatric Institute Research Program, Camarillo, California.

LUKE S. WATSON, JR., Ph.D.: Behavior Modification Technology, Inc., Libertyville, Illinois.

PREFACE

T HIS BOOK GREW out of a symposium of the same name presented at the annual convention of the Association for the Advancement of Behavior Therapy (AABT) in New York City, during October 1972. This symposium, in turn, was suggested by the efforts of a number of us beginning in October of 1970 to create a behavior therapy program on a state hospital ward which utilized token economy methods as one form of treatment. Naturally enough, this effort began with reviewing much of the published literature. We also had the advantage of visiting token economies in operation in the Los Angeles area and the obtaining of expert advice from such people as Doctors Tom Ball, Pat Martin, Jackie Montgomery, H. H. Schaefer, and others. It became apparent that there are a number of ways of solving the routine problems of token economy operation. These problems are relatively minor in the sense that they do not pose any major theoretical questions nor do they necessarily involve any new methods of behavioral change; but they are of major importance in another respect because they *must* be solved in order to create and maintain an effective token economy. However, few books have been published in this area.

Since these matters troubled us, we surmised that they must also bother others working with the problems of starting and maintaining effective token systems. The response given to the AABT symposium demonstrated that we were correct. The attendance was standing room only, and even that was exhausted. The program was scheduled to last for one and one-half hours, but the discussion prompted by questions from the audience extended the length to three hours and ten minutes; finally the chairman (the editor) terminated it. It would seem that these matters are of considerable concern to a number of people.

In creating this book, the editor asked the original symposium presenters to expand upon their previous, rather brief presentations and to include their most current thinking on these matters. All but one of the original contributors (Dr. E. McInnis) wrote chapters for this book. In addition, other knowledgeable persons consented to contribute (Drs. Luke Watson, John Foreyt, and Charles Wallace; Val Baker and John Davis). The editor sincerely hopes that the assembled material serves to assist others in their efforts to create and *maintain* useful behavior modification programs.

ROGER L. PATTERSON

CONTENTS

MAINTAINING EFFECTIVE
TOKEN ECONOMIES

Chapter I

INTRODUCTION

ROGER L. PATTERSON, PH.D.

THIS BOOK IS written for those who are already familiar with the basic principles utilized in token economies as explained by Ayllon and Azrin (1968), Atthowe and Krasner (1968), Schaefer and Martin (1969), and others. The purpose of this book is not to explain the basic principles, but rather to provide the reader with answers to some of the problems which it is necessary to solve in order to established and especially to *maintain* an effective therapy program which utilizes token economy methodology.

In order to accomplish this purpose, a number of experienced and successful practitioners in the field were presented with some specific questions which, the editor felt, have to be answered by anyone who manages a token economy. These were the following:

1. How should line staff be selected to work in a token economy?
2. How should staff be trained?
3. How should token economy programs be designed to provide for individualized treatment programs?
4. What are some ways to communicate treatment information to *all* staff who interact with the patient?
5. What methods allow for the collection of diversified but reliable data?
6. How does one design data and program information systems to allow for sufficiently frequent and rapid revisions?
7. How is frequent and appropriate staff reinforcement accomplished?

The above questions are not the only ones that one could raise about successful token economy operations; however, answers to them must be found by the token economy manager who wishes to have a lasting program which produces changes in human behavior.

No contributor to this book was asked to provide answers to all of these questions. The authors were free to select some of them to answer. However, all the authors were asked to draw upon their experience and their knowledge of relevant literature in providing solutions to these problems which have been demonstrated to be *practical*. This is intended to be a book for the practitioner who wishes to use the experience and empirical findings of others in solving some of his own difficulties in the management of his or her token programs.

Just as all the contributors did not answer all the questions, several of the contributors answered the same questions in different ways. The editor feels that this is highly desirable, as one of the purposes of the book is to provide the reader with several *alternative* approaches to the proposed questions. There are also instances in which the points emphasized by some authors are remarkably similar. While it might have simplified matters for the editor and the publisher to call these similarities "overlap" and thus to delete them, this would be against the purpose of this book by not allowing each author to give his own ideas about the problems under consideration. Instances of such concurrence of opinion may be regarded by the reader as votes of confidence for the point at hand.

It can be argued that there is an empirically "best" answer to each of the proposed questions. However, the reader will see in the systems described herein, that target populations, institutional settings, administrative policies, type of staff available, budget, and other situational variables make it impossible (perhaps unfortunately) for anyone to devise an empirically based "ideal" token economy which can then be replicated by all. Establishing a token economy will probably always remain an engineering problem in which empirically based principles are used to devise situationally specific applications.

In the first article, Kazdin has drawn heavily upon his extensive knowledge of the empirical behavior modification literature. He concentrates much of his effort on the training of staff and on procedures employed to maintain staff performance. He also includes considerable discussion on the appropriate role of the staff and also the role of the patients in carrying out the operations of the token economy. While some authors (see the chapter by Patterson) maintain that maximum individualization of treatment is desirable, Kazdin presents evidence that group contingencies have been highly effective in some cases.

McInnis also chose to concentrate on staff training and management. However, his approach is different from Kazdin's in that he has integrated methods and ideas used in business management and forms of therapy other than token economy into his planning.

The papers by Kazdin and McInnis are the most general in the sense that they discuss the literature more extensively. The rest of the chapters are more specific in the sense that they concentrate more on particular methodologies and ideas which the authors found to be useful in their own work.

Watson's approach is somewhat radical in that he advocates reorganizing the entire institution to be consistent with a "rehabilitation orientation as opposed to a custodial treatment orientation" in order to effect an efficient system of behavioral change. One might infer from his writing that he seems to be saying, "Don't fight the system, change it." There is considerable merit in this point of view; however, changing institutional management systems can sometimes be prohibitively difficult. Watson makes the very cogent point that the entire management structure of the institution should be dictated by an analysis of the specific objectives of changing the behavior of the population. The methods of providing for staff training, staff accountability, and staff reinforcement described by Watson should be read by anyone in this field. This chapter also presents some original ideas with regard to reinforcing appropriate behavior in nontreatment and administrative staff, a matter to which too little attention is given.

While Watson says large institutions should be drastically changed, Patterson says that we should get out of such places to do our treatment. He uses his experience in two small, intensive treatment settings to make the point that people originally come to treatment for highly idiosyncratic behaviors. It is only when we herd them together in large institutions that we come to view human treatment as a mass production problem. Patterson argues, by presenting examples of two highly individualized programs, that it is desirable and possible to attend to each individual's needs on an individual basis.

Chapter VI of this book, by Wallace, et al. follows Patterson's for two reasons. Wallace, et al. present a method for easily individualizing the assignment of routine ward jobs and the collection of individual performance data for these jobs. This method could easily be applied to larger settings. This system for routine jobs is combined with other systems to maintain completely individualized treatment. In addition to the individualization aspect, the chapters by Patterson and Wallace, et al. are of interest for another reason. Wallace became Program Director of the Clinical Research Unit at Camarillo State Hospital (California) immediately after Patterson resigned from this position. The description of the development of this experimental treatment center provides a rare opportunity to show how a token economy can, and should, continue to develop and refine its techniques.

Atthowe describes the long-term development of one of the earlier token economies. The emphasis of this program has been on achieving shaping for large numbers of individuals by means of categorizing them according to their behavioral accomplishments (a "levels" system). In effect, more achievement produces more desirable reinforcers. Consistent with the policy of this book, Atthowe does not go into great detail in explaining this program, as the basics have been published earlier. Rather, he presents a summary description of the earlier work and then goes on to explain the later efforts to extend the "levels" concept to life outside the hospital. As Atthowe notes, it is the ability of our programs to produce changes in the behavior of people in the natural environment which will ultimately determine our success.

Foreyt begins by emphasizing, in agreement with other authors, that it is necessary to have complete cooperation of the administration in order to effectively run a token economy. He then presents a particular data system utilizing "punch cards," which he says permits greater contingency control and more manageable data collection on the ward. He also presents some data indicating that his program has long-term effects.

The reader is invited to compare and contrast the ideas and methodologies presented above. The editor considers this a wealth of practical information, and he sincerely wishes that he had had this information at hand when he first began his efforts to create a token economy. Hopefully, others will benefit.

REFERENCES

Atthowe, J. M., Jr., and Krasner, L.: Preliminary report on the application of contingent reinforcement procedure (token economy) on a "chronic" psychiatric ward. *J Abnorm Psychol*, 73:37, 1968.

Ayllon, T., and Azrin, N. H.: *The Token Economy: A Motivational System for Therapy and Rehabilitation*. New York, Appleton, 1968.

Shaefer, H. H., and Martin, P. L.: *Behavioral Therapy*. New York, McGraw, 1969.

Chapter II

IMPLEMENTING TOKEN PROGRAMS: THE USE OF STAFF AND PATIENTS FOR MAXIMIZING CHANGE

Alan E. Kazdin, Ph.D.

Implementing token economies in psychiatric settings, and other settings as well, requires resolution of a variety of issues and obstacles. Particular concern has been voiced over issues pertaining to training ward staff, utilizing the staff in the token program, the types of contingencies which can be used for the patients, and the relative merits of such contingencies. In the present paper, several issues which will be discussed include improving staff performance on the ward, expanding the tasks in the program that both staff and patients perform, and developing contingencies in the hospital to increase patients' responsiveness to their social environment. The paper will emphasize practical solutions as well as research findings for resolving issues encountered in implementing token programs.

STAFF TRAINING

A highly trained staff is essential in administering a token economy. Because the primary goal of the token program is to alter patient behavior, staff training is often given only a cursory treatment. Admittedly, a few token programs have been effective without elaborate staff training (e.g. Christopherson, et al., 1972). Yet such programs are not conducted in institutional

Preparation of this paper was facilitated, in part, by a grant from the National Institute of Mental Health (MH 23399).

settings where a wide range of behaviors and a large number of clients often are incorporated into the contingencies.

Although providing adequate staff training is a formidable task, it introduces no new problems for the behavior modifier. In fact, all of the problems attendant upon developing behaviors with the patients occur in advance with the staff. Target behaviors need to be carefully defined, data needs to be gathered on these behaviors, a specific program need to be implemented, the efficacy of the program needs to be demonstrated, and maintenance of staff behavior needs to be programmed. In spite of the symmetry in the tasks required for staff and patient change, the literature reveals a gross asymmetry in the procedures used to effect these changes. Nevertheless, a number of techniques have been employed to train attendants and aides.

Training Techniques

Instructional Techniques

Instructional methods including lectures, discussions, workshops, in-service training, and course work frequently are used to train staff in behavior modification techniques. In most cases, the efficacy of these procedures is not evaluated. Instructional techniques have taken many forms. Yet the results are reasonably consistent. When psychiatric attendants are merely instructed to behave in a particular way *vis à vis* the patients (i.e. reinforce certain behavior), there is virtually no change in the staff behavior (Katz, et al., 1972). Even if staff are given constant reminders on the ward to use reinforcement (Katz, et al., 1972), or are encouraged to interact with their patients (Pomerleau, et al., 1973), their behavior is largely unaffected.

Instructional methods sometimes consist of planned lectures and discussions off the ward. While lectures and discussions provide staff with knowledge of the principles of behavior modification, they do not train proficiency in actually carrying out the procedures (Gardner, 1972). Didactic procedures have documented efficacy with hospital staff if they are supplemented with applied training on the ward (Paul, et al., 1973). As a minimal requirement, staff training programs which rely on instructional techniques should supplement training with practice either on the ward or in simulated role-playing situations to ensure that staff can execute the contingencies. Generally, instructional methods used alone are ineffective in training staff.

Feedback

Feedback refers to providing staff with information regarding the adequacy of their performance. For many individuals, feedback operates as a conditioned reinforcer. While feedback is inherent in virtually all forms of response consequation (e.g. delivery of praise, tokens, reprimands), it can be used independently of these other events.

Feedback has not been evaluated extensively in training institutional staff. In one program, attendants received classroom training to develop self-help skills in retarded residents (Panyan, et al., 1970). Staff were responsible for conducting sessions using operant techniques with the residents. Initially, consequences for the staff were not associated with conducting or failing to conduct resident training sessions. A feedback procedure was implemented which consisted of providing staff with a "feedback sheet." The sheet indicated the percentage of sessions conducted by a staff member out of all possible opportunities. Staff increased the number of sessions with the residents when the feedback procedure was used. Similarly, informing psychiatric aides about the progress of their patients relative to the patients of other aides altered staff performance (Pomerleau, et al., 1973).

Most investigations employing feedback as a staff training technique have been conducted in schools to train teachers. Typically, verbal or written feedback is provided. Feedback delivered in the classroom while the teacher is interacting with the students or after school has been effective in some cases but not in others (Breyer and Allen, 1972; Cooper, et al., 1970; Cossairt, et al., 1973). In general, feedback has not been the most effective technique in altering staff behavior.

Social Reinforcement

Praise, approval, and attention have not been systematically evaluated as techniques to train hospital attendants and aides in behavior modification. Yet, praise has been useful in training individuals in noninstitutional settings to employ behavior modification techniques. For example, contingent praise has been used to increase teachers' use of reinforcement with their students (Brown, et al., 1969; Cossairt, et al., 1973). Positive comments by staff who supervise attendants or administrators might be highly effective if delivered contingently for staff performance.

Token Reinforcement

Tangible conditioned reinforcers have been used effectively in a number of instances to train institutional staff. Bricker, et al. (1972) provided video feedback to attendants for their performance on the ward. While staff viewed themselves on tape, they received verbal praise and trading stamps from the project director. The reinforcers were contingent upon staff interacting with the residents (as recorded on tape). The contingency increased staff-resident interaction on the ward by 700 percent relative to baseline. The changes were attributed primarily to reinforcement because removal of feedback did not result in a decrease in the target behavior.

Katz, et al. (1972) demonstrated that contingent cash bonuses increased the use of reinforcement of psychiatric staff and increased task-oriented (work) behavior of the patients. Other investigators have shown the effect of monetary reinforcement in changing staff behavior using the behavior of the clients they supervise as the criterion for staff reinforcement (Pomerleau, et al., 1972; Pomerleau, et al., 1973). Typically, staff are told they will receive a monetary bonus for increasing their use of reinforcement with the patients. As might be expected, merely giving extra money to staff is not sufficient to alter their behavior. Only when the monetary reinforcement is contingent upon specific behaviors does staff behavior reliably change (Pomerleau, et al., 1973).

Modeling

Modeling has not been used frequently as a technique to train institutional staff in behavior modification. Modeling may be quite useful as a training technique because individuals can readily acquire complex behaviors through observation. Staff members undergoing training often note that the training is distant from the actual situation on the ward. Thus, it might be useful for an expert to administer the contingencies and demonstate the techniques in the actual situation in which the staff function.

A recent study attests to the efficacy of modeling in training behavior modification skills. In a classroom situation, a trained behavior modifier initially conducted a token reinforcement program in the presence of the teacher (Ringer, 1973). In a short time, the experimenter (model) gradually allowed the teacher to assume increasingly greater responsibility for the program. Eventually, the experimenter left the classroom and the teacher maintained the program. Although child behavior was slightly better when the experimenter was involved in the program, inappropriate child behavior was maintained at a low rate relative to baseline after he had left.

In one hospital, a psychologist served as a model for the staff by providing a daily demonstration of reinforcement with a difficult patient. This procedure did not result in substantial effects on staff, at least as indirectly assessed through patient improvements (Pomerleau, et al., 1973).

Training: General Comments

In any staff training program, data need to be collected to evaluate the procedures. Evaluation of staff performance, as of the clients', is essential. Only with careful demonstration can the staff be considered trained. Training is not defined by the procedures to which staff are exposed but by the changes in behavior resulting from such exposure.

Evaluation needs to include all, or at least most, of the behaviors that training is designed to alter (Kazdin, 1973b). It cannot be assumed that altering one or a few behaviors will generalize to other responses. Evidence suggests that only those specific behaviors trained are altered and not related responses which would make the staff more effective behavioral engineers

(Cooper, et al., 1970). Moreover, if a response is trained to be executed only a few times during the day, it may not generalize to nontrained times during the same days (Fielding, et al., 1971). If the goals of training include changes in several staff behaviors, which are performed at several times or in various situations, training has to include the range of exigencies.

The goals of staff training include long-term changes in staff behavior. Hence, training must provide a means whereby staff behavior remains at a consistently high level of competence. However, too little data are collected to ensure that the initial goals of training have been achieved, to say nothing of follow-up information. Often it is assumed that once staff behaviors are developed, they will be maintained at a high level. The putative "natural contingencies" are expected to maintain staff behaviors. These natural events refer to the increased effectiveness the staff will have on the patients which will reinforce staff behavior. However, it has been well demonstrated that as soon as extrinsic consequences for staff behavior are withdrawn, behavior reverts to pretraining levels (Katz, et al., 1972; Panyan, et al., 1970; Pomerleau, et al., 1973).

Practical Considerations

In practice, it is difficult to conduct an elaborate training program despite the primary importance of such an endeavor. There are several reasons for this. First, it is difficult to monitor staff behavior on the ward to evaluate the training techniques. Evaluation of staff behavior is personally odious to many staff members. Surveillance of staff may result in undesirable reactions to the training program. A possible solution is to evaluate the efficacy of staff training on the behavior of the residents (e.g. Pomerleau, et al., 1973). When the patients' behavior changes, this is perfectly adequate as an indirect measure of training. However, sometimes staff behavior may change but not sufficiently to produce a noticeable difference in the client's behavior. Further, a given contingency, even if implemented correctly, may not change a patient's behavior (Kazdin, 1973a). In such cases, evaluation of patient behavior might be mistakenly interpreted as a failure of staff to carry out the program properly. Direct observation of both staff and patient behavior is the best procedure for evaluating staff training.

In cases where it is not feasible to observe staff behavior, staff can record their own responses. Of course, self-monitoring has its own problems, such as obtaining reliability of the monitored data (Kazdin, 1974). Yet, in difficult situations where other resources are not available, self-monitoring with some reliability checks is vastly superior to no data collection.

A second issue of practical concern is identifying sources of reinforcement that can be used during and subsequent to formal staff training. Although many reinforcers come to mind, such as vacations, bonuses, work-shift preferences, time-off work, raises, and promotions, these have been used in relatively few programs. In most institutions, these rewards are not readily available for delivery contingent upon desirable staff performance, as defined by the program coordinators. Nevertheless, there are many reinforcers which can be used. Contingent recognition of the attendants' achievements can reinforce staff behavior. Some programs designate a staff member of the month (Roberts and Perry, 1970). Certificates or letters of commendation can be placed in the staff member's file contingent upon desirable performance. Feedback can also be used. Patterson, et al. (1972) employed a weekly feedback newsletter to staff which summarizes patients' progress and comments on achievements by staff. Feedback can also be delivered in the form of graphs of patient changes. Since feedback tends to have variable effects on staff, other sources of staff reinforcement probably need to be sought.

Caution is required in using some reinforcers. In some cases, union requirements militate against using work-related reinforcers and discriminating among staff (i.e. selectively dispensing the reinforcers). Further, providing extra reinforcers to individuals who are working well may lead to resentment by those who do not earn them. Unless an individualized staff training program is devised, it is usually those staff members whose behavior is already adequate who earn the reinforcers. If those staff whose behavioral skills are weak are selected as targets of a staff behavior modification program, this too may be received with resentment. Administering reinforcers to the staff may require consideration of more interpersonal exigencies than do programs of the patients. Selection of reinforcers, evaluation of performance, and control over other available reinforcers (including escape) are more restricted with the staff than with the patients.

RESISTANCE ON THE PART OF THE STAFF

There has been a great deal of concern with resistance and negative attitudes on the part of staff. Unfortunately, there has been relatively little research on staff attitude and its relation to staff and patient behavior. In one project, it was noted that staff attitude across two wards covaried with program efficacy (Suchotliff, et al., 1970). Staff on the ward where the token program was effective were less custodial in their orientation than staff on the ward where the program had no effect. These results do not imply that initially favorable attitudes necessarily result in significant staff attitude change (McReynolds and Coleman, 1972). Nevertheless, staff attitude may be an important variable worth evaluating.

Initial resistance on the part of staff should come as no surprise. Rarely do attendants select behavior modification as a treatment modality, but have the techniques imposed upon them (e.g. after the institution receives a grant). Moreover, staff frequently fail to recognize that they will actually receive much help on the ward in changing the problems as they perceive them. Training may seem unrelated to the problems staff encounter. Operant principles, the importance of data collection, exigencies of single subject designs, and related topics are discussed and perhaps appreciated but are not sufficiently concrete to many staff members.

Attempts should be made to alter any initial staff resistance to the program. Poor attitudes may be manifest in verbal operants, but may embrace other behaviors as well, such as the manner in which reinforcement is delivered. Various means of overcoming negative evaluations could be incorporated into staff training. Research on attitude change suggests means which may be used. For example, role playing, particularly when the role enactments are improvised by the individual, effectively alters attitudes. For staff on the ward, designing and implementing programs provide opportunities for such role play and improvisation. A staff member who plays an integral part in the program is less likely to disparage that program than one whose role is less significant. Even where staff attitude change is not a primary target, staff should be invested as much as possible with responsibility for the program. It is of less consequence if someone else's program is not executed properly than if one's own is not. The selection of staff-designed programs can be used as a reinforcer for staff performance. Staff who meet certain performance criteria could be reinforced by implementing a program in which they have had a major part in constructing.

Training staff whose behavior is "negativistic" may begin as a shaping task for the psychologist. For example, many staff members initially find the collection of data repugnant. Despite acknowledging the possible value of objective evaluative measures, the procedures hardly seem worth the effort. Initially, small and reasonable demands can be made upon the staff. The demands will vary depending upon the staff member who is to be trained. Some members may start by collecting data for two or three fifteen-minute periods in a forty-hour week. Indeed, staff who show some hesitation in collecting data can be queried as to the amount of time they would be willing to devote to collecting information. After any data are collected, the psychologist can reinforce steps which increasingly approximate the final data-collection format.

Initial observation by the staff can be directed toward their own behavior. This may be useful for three reasons: (1) Observation of oneself is sufficiently interesting to many to encourage observation; (2) many individuals are surprised at the data provided from self-observation; and (3) self-observation sometimes is very reactive. It may effect sufficient changes in staff behavior to achieve therapeutic ends for the client (e.g. Herbert and Baer, 1972). On other occasions, staff recognize that their behavior may have some relation to that of the patient. Of course, the potential benefits of self-observation are side effects. The main purpose is to shape "data-collecting" behavior.

ADMINISTRATIVE SUPPORT

Support for the program at administrative levels has obvious importance. Decisions in the institutions can be made to interfere with the program, including transfer of staff or patients to different wards, not allowing use of specific reinforcers, interfering with exigencies of experimental evaluation of the program, among others (Hall and Baker, 1973). There seems to be no research, at least in token economies, which provides techniques to resolve the problems encountered at administrative levels.

Developing support (whatever this might be behaviorally) in administrators may be an important aspect of staff training at some institutions. To enhance support, it is desirable to have administrative input for the program in terms of patient target behaviors and selection of contingencies from the available and sound alternatives. Providing input for the program is likely to increase administrative involvement. Administrators also wish their clientele to be helped, but are rarely allowed an active role in this process. Usually, it is not difficult to obtain input from administrators, when programs for the patients are being designed.

Another important feature in obtaining administrative support is constantly reporting the results of the program to the administrators. Most institutional treatment programs do not provide rigorous data which attest to their efficacy. This is unfortunate for a number of reasons. Even when rigorous data are available, they are rarely presented to administrative staff. Typically, the data resulting from operant programs is compelling. Results often are clear and dramatic and speak for themselves. If the results pertain to problems in which an administrator is interested, they can be all the more potent in fostering support. In most cases, clear data, even if not indicative of behavior change in a given patient, are noteworthy against the usual background of nonevaluated programs.

UTILIZATION OF STAFF AND PATIENTS

Role of the Staff

The primary task for attendants is implementing the contingencies and collecting data to evaluate these contingencies. This role certainly is a more significant contribution to treatment than the custodial role traditionally accorded ward staff. Yet staff should be directly involved in program planning, including isolating target behaviors and recommending contingencies, rather than simply implementing programs in which they play little or no part in designing. The staff involvement in planning should be as great as their training and capabilities allow, culminating in the design of programs. There are several reasons for this strategy beyond aggrandizement of attendants.

In most institutions, serving as an aide provides minimal reinforcers. Praise, prestige, status, money, and rewards of recognizing therapeutic progress are usually foreign to aide and attendant status. Custodial behavior on the part of hospital attendants is sometimes decried as an unfortunate plot contrived by the staff, rather than a function of the environment in which such staff behaviors are systematically, albeit inadvertently, shaped (Ullmann, 1967). There are contingencies which foster an "aide culture" both in terms of selection of initial candidates for employment and for consequation of the behaviors in the institution. A major contributing factor to custodial behavior may be that progress on the part of the patients is rarely achieved and perhaps not even sought. Custodial behaviors on the part of staff often meet implicit institutional demands for patient care.

One major change which is readily feasible is the elevation in status and responsibility of the job which aides and attendants perform. The status and responsibility of the staff can be increased by providing staff with skills to design and evaluate the behavioral programs rather than merely to implement them. One possible benefit of such an approach with aides may be to decrease employee turnover. Further, the staff attracted to a position specifically outlined as supervisory rather than custodial may include personnel whose propensities toward or interest in custodial behaviors may be lower due to factors of selection.

The demands of supervision and program evaluation require greater training than custodial care. Staff members need to achieve a different level of training than is normally achieved with staff training programs (Gardner, 1973). If the role of staff is enhanced by adding responsibility, delimiting custodial activities, and training more complex activities such as designing and evaluating programs, an obvious question arises. Who will implement the actual contingencies on the ward which ordinarily are administered by the staff? The answer certainly is not unique and has precedence in the token economy literature, at least on a small scale.

Role of the Patients

Limiting implementation of the contingencies to available staff precludes utilization of a potentially large available source of manpower, *viz.* the patients. The patients themselves can be involved directly in the management of the token economy. While some programs have involved patients in activities, such as running a ward canteen, collecting tokens for activities, and working the token "bank," several other activities are available which may be more directly related to the implementation of the contingencies. Patients might be able to monitor their own contingencies or those of others, gather data, design new contingencies for the ward as a whole, and determine future program directions. Some attempts to utilize patients in staff functions have been made. In a few programs patients are partially responsible for smooth running of the ward. Some patients are in charge of supervising work assignments on the ward (e.g. Heap, et al., 1970). Also, in one program, a ward "police force" made up of patients served to quell physical violence and to follow instructions from staff in times of disorders (Pomerleau, et al., 1972). Patient positions of responsibility on the ward usually are reinforced with extra tokens. With nonpsychiatric populations, clients have been relied upon extensively to deliver reinforcement to their peers or participate in response consequation in some way (e.g. Solomon and Wahler, 1973).

Involving the clients themselves in execution of their own contingencies may have beneficial effects on behavior (Kazdin,

1973a). For example, with children, performance is sometimes greater under self-imposed token reinforcement contingencies than under externally imposed contingencies (Lovitt and Curtiss, 1969). In hospital settings, investigators have reported the use of clients in their own reinforcement program (e.g. Olson and Greenberg, 1972).

Utilizing patients in functions typically reserved for staff offers several potential advantages. First, personnel are placed in a role of supervising patients which allows staff to oversee and direct a larger number of programs than if they were the sole dispensers of token reinforcement. Second, staff cannot always monitor the behavior that takes place when a group is relatively unsupervised or when staff-patient ratios are small. When reinforcement contingencies are administered solely by the staff, the problem of patient surveillance becomes acute. The patients themselves can monitor their own behavior and that of their peers on more occasions than staff and across a larger number of situations. Third, if only staff are used to reinforce desirable behavior, they are likely to exert stimulus control over that behavior. Clients make subtle discriminations across individuals who administer reinforcement differently (Redd, 1969).

Performance and consequation in the presence of peers on the ward may be different from performance in the presence of staff. It is no surprise that an anecdotal report from one program indicated that paranoid ideation occurred in the presence of staff but not in their absence (i.e. between patients) (cf. Liberman, 1968). The stimulus control by staff can interfere with the long-range goals of generalization of performance across a wide range of people. Generalization may be achieved more readily by utilizing the patients in addition to staff for reinforcement of target behaviors.

INDIVIDUALIZED AND GROUP CONTINGENCIES

In designing a token economy, a major issue is whether the contingencies for the patients should be individualized or based upon group performance. There are a variety of types of contingencies included in each of these categories. The practical feasibility and advantages in terms of patient behavior change differ across types of contingencies.

Individualized contingencies usually refer to performance criteria and consequences which are suited to a particular patient's behavior. Contingencies can be individualized along different dimensions, such as the target behavior, the performance criteria for the target behavior, the consequences, and the parameters of consequence delivery, including magnitude, schedule, and delay of the consequence. At one end of the continuum of individualization, each patient on a ward can be reinforced for a different behavior (e.g. grooming for one patient and reading for another patient), receive different consequences for the behavior (e.g. overnight pass or access to TV), and earn the consequence on different schedules (e.g. at the end of a week or daily). Less individualization is apparent in contingencies where several individuals are reinforced for a given behavior (e.g. grooming) and receive identical consequences (e.g. a particular reinforcer). Individualization here refers to criterion for earning the reinforcer which differs across individuals. The ease with which individualized contingencies can be implemented depends in a large measure on the degree of individualization which is sought (i.e. the number of dimensions along which the individual contingencies vary).

Group contingencies also refer to a variety of operations. One way to structure group contingencies is to allow the behavior of the group as a whole to dictate the consequence earned by each individual. In this procedure, a criterion of performance for the group is set. Only if the criterion is achieved is the reinforcer earned. Each individual is reinforced if the group achieves some criterion. For example, a group of patients might earn an overnight pass if there are no infractions of ward rules by any patient for one week. A second way to use a group contingency is to adhere to the same criterion for response consequation for each member of the group. The performance of the individual must meet a standard criterion (e.g. making one's bed), if the individual is to earn the consequence. Yet, the earning of a consequence of a given individual is independent of earning by other individuals.

Practical Considerations

The differences in individual and group contingencies are not merely academic. At the practical level, there are several considerations dictating the selection of the type of contingency employed. Individualized contingencies, obviously, are prohibitive on a large scale. Staff resources ordinarily are quite limited. Thus, in most institutions, the gains of establishing extensively individualized programs have to be evaluated against the losses of including relatively few patients in the program. If staff resources are supplemented with assistance from the patients in implementing the program and monitoring the contingencies, reliance upon individualized contingencies can be augmented greatly.

Another consideration in using individualized versus group contingencies is the heterogeneity of the patients. Patients with similar target behaviors can readily be placed into group contingencies. Indeed, in most programs target behaviors are selected to be trained ward-wide (e.g. self-care and social skills). Group contingencies usually are required for some behaviors because institutionalized patients have (or perhaps develop as part of their institutionalization) a certain number of homogeneous problems. Group contingencies are well suited to problems of reasonably wide generality.

In deciding whether to use group or individualized contingencies, it is tempting to sacrifice significance of the focus of the program for ease of application. For example, in some institutions, programs are developed for those behaviors which have wide generality, albeit behavior change in these areas is of dubious value. The convenience of group contingencies allows hospitals to implement programs on a large scale. For many institutions, administrative pressure contributes to a focus on the number of patients in the program rather than social significance of the behavior to be changed and the impact of change on any given patient.

In many programs, group and individualized contingencies are combined in some way. One way to combine individualized and group contingencies is to employ levelled token systems. In such a system, patients are grouped into various levels or steps in the program (Kazdin and Bootzin, 1972) according to performance criteria (e.g. token earnings) and rate of improvement. Deindividualization is achieved in at least two ways in a levelled system. First, at each level there are certain behaviors which must be performed before progressing to higher levels. Further, the reinforcers available usually are determined by the level in which the individual is placed. Even though individuals are grouped, individualized criteria for performance can be included in the contingency requirements for progression into higher levels. For example, patients may have to decrease their "symptomatic" behavior or other idiosyncracies before progressing. Since these behaviors differ across patients, the contingencies, to some extent at least, are individualized. Yet, the main organization of the system is in groups.

A second way to incorporate group contingencies along with individual contingencies is to employ consequence sharing. In consequence sharing, the behavior of one individual dictates the reinforcers (or aversive events) which are earned by the group. Typically, one individual earns the reinforcers but the reinforcers are divided among the peers (e.g. Wolf, et al., 1970).

Reinforcer sharing can also be based upon the performance of a small group of individuals or indeed, as mentioned earlier, the group as a whole. However, when consequences earned by a single individual are shared, the criteria for reinforcement are individualized. The group portion of the contingency only refers to how the social situation is structured to support that individual's behavior. Yet, there is a group contingency also operative. The group receives reinforcers for a given individual's performance. Thus, for the group to be reinforced, members must engage in specific behaviors such as prompting the behavior of the target subject and providing social consequences.

Treatment Considerations

It is sometimes assumed that individualization of contingencies is an ideal toward which all institutions should strive. There is no doubt that individualized focus is ideal from several standpoints mentioned earlier. However, group or ward-wide contingencies have led to dramatic changes in psychiatric patients as well as other groups (Kazdin, 1975). Thus, a number of token programs have shown improvements with group programs with relatively little individualization of the contingencies. Some research suggests group and individual contingencies are not differentially effective (e.g. Axelrod, 1973). However, in a program for a given individual, evidence suggests that using the group for reinforcer sharing results in greater behavior change than that achieved without group participation (e.g. Wolf, et al., 1970).

There are additional treatment considerations in using contingencies which involve the group. There are problems peculiar to a large institution which may make the setting undesirable for rehabilitation. Individualized treatment programs alone may not remedy this. In a typical institution general contingencies need to be provided to overcome possible deleterious effects of institutionalization. In addition to focusing on particular patients, some efforts are required for ward-wide programs. In a sense, some general contingencies may be needed to overcome the effects of the setting itself. For other reasons, group contingencies may make a significant contribution to a patient's rehabilitation. Group contingencies of various kinds may be useful in relating a patient's behavior to the group. For example, in one program (Pomerleau, et al., 1972) patients were organized into dyads, and dyads organized into polydyads. A patient's infraction of a ward rule resulted in a fine for both the patient and his dyad partner. Relatively flagrant fines resulted in each polydyad member paying for the infraction by the individual. In another program (Olson & Greenberg, 1972), group performance partially determined whether reinforcers would be available to individual patients. The ward was divided into four groups of patients. One reinforcer in the system was a patient's access to his own personal funds (or coupons negotiable at a canteen). However, whether a patient could receive reinforcers was determined not only by his performance but also by the performance of the group to which he belonged. The types of group contingencies in these programs presumably help train patients to monitor the behaviors of others who might influence their own fate as well as control their own behaviors which can influence the fate of others. While the contingencies are group contingencies, they allow for individualization of criteria for response consequation. For psychiatric patients the combination of group and individualized contingencies is probably the most profitable not only for staff convenience but more importantly for patients' socialization. Certainly, empirical work is required to evaluate the effects of group and individualized contingencies on patient and staff performance.

COMMUNICATION AND EXECUTION OF THE CONTINGENCIES

Effectively communicating individualized patient programs to ward personnel is a difficult job, particularly if the experimental conditions are being "reversed" or modified to evaluate the contingencies, or if individualized programs are constantly changing in response to patient progress. There is a need for consistency in the patient contingencies, especially in the initial stages of a program. Communication may be handled differently depending upon where information problems arise.

Communication may be problematic with staff of the token economy ward (e.g. between different shifts) or with staff who have little contact with the patients (e.g. from different wards). On the behavioral ward there should be little difficulty in keeping staff informed about individualized programs. Several procedures can be used to enhance communication, such as frequent meetings, program summaries placed on bulletin boards (which all attendants might be required to initial each day), and newsletters which extend information to the staff on the ward. Those individuals on the ward who have major responsibility for the patients are relatively easily informed of existing practices. The problem in staff communication on the ward may be evident when personnel design or inadvertently execute conflicting programs so that one attendant attends to bizarre behaviors while another ignores them, or when different definitions of target behaviors are used for reinforcement (Ayllon and Azrin, 1968).

In discussing communication of programs to staff, a distinction should be made between staff knowledge and performance. It is often assumed that if staff are equally informed of the contingencies, they will execute them in the same fashion. This remains only an assumption in most programs. There may be a problem on the ward which might be referred to as *contingency inconsistency*. This simply means that as contingencies are executed, there may be gross discrepancies across staff members or within individual members over time (Ayllon and Azrin, 1968; Suchotliff, et al., 1970).

In behavior modification programs it is common practice to obtain reliability checks between observers on the target behaviors to ensure that these responses are monitored with high levels of agreement. Interobserver agreement is usually regarded as essential. In contrast, agreement between staff members in administering the contingency is rarely required. Even where staff are the observers as well as reinforcing agents, agreement, if documented, usually is emphasized as part of the data collection rather than as part of the administration of the contingencies. Reliability between ward staff needs to be estimated periodically to ensure that consequences for patient performance are delivered for the same response requirements. Staff can be checked intermittently to rate how many tokens should be given for particular behaviors. (Videotape replay of various patient behaviors might facilitate this.) Discrepancies in staff performance will provide impetus for clarification in administering the program. Effective communication of programs on the ward entails much more than disseminating information on individualized programs. Although such dissemination is a prerequisite, interstaff consistency in the execution of the contingencies is crucial. Similarly, intra-individual consistency over time must be monitored to ensure that a given attendant does not change.

Ayllon and Azrin (1968) emphasize the importance of staff consistency. In designing programs, they recommend adherence to the Direct Supervision Rule, *viz.* provide systematic and direct observation of the execution of the reinforcement procedure (p. 145). Performance can be monitored on a variable schedule so as not to consume an extensive amount of supervising time.

Ayllon and Azrin point to numerous instances in which staff inconsistently administered contingencies which, of course, would not have been detected had no direct supervision of reinforcement exchange been programmed into the system.

Outside of communication among staff on the ward, a great problem is communicating programs to personnel not in frequent contact with the patient. One must ask how desirable or essential such communication is for all personnel interacting with the patient. In most programs, it would not seem essential that personnel know the precise contingencies which constitute a particular patient's program. If personnel have general skills and guidelines, their overall performance should not interfere with the program's efficacy. There is no substitute for dealing with a patient consistently on and off the ward. A number of programs have been with chronic patients whose activities off the ward are minimal. Perhaps as more programs are developed with fewer chronic patients in an open ward (where free access to the entire grounds is mandatory), off-ward staff will assume a greater role.

To communicate with staff off the ward, the patient can carry a card wherever he goes in the hospital. The card can include categories of behavior such as social responses, grooming, and work behaviors which are codified. Personnel coming in contact with the patient can peruse the card and determine those areas focused upon on the ward. This can at least inform staff, otherwise unfamiliar with the program, to avoid potentially conflicting treatment prescriptions or interactions related to the target areas.

As the initial goals of a program are achieved, the patient needs to learn to respond consistently to individuals who are not necessarily continuing the ward contingencies. Valuable information can be obtained from individuals in contact with the patient who are not carrying out or are not even aware of the program. The cost required in training off-ward staff on a systematic basis and subsequently monitoring their behavior is prohibitive for most institutions. This situation is not to be lamented. Complete control of all the contingencies may not be essential to effect rehabilitation.

CONCLUDING COMMENTS

A variety of practical problems arise in conducting any treatment program in an institutional setting. The requirements for implementing and evaluating token economies or any other behavior modification program are somewhat more demanding than for many other procedures. Many traditional approaches have not permitted treatment to leave the hands of trained professionals. Hence, the issue of training attendants and aides is less relevant. In contrast, staff who administer a behavior modification program are crucial in effecting therapeutic change. Thus, careful staff training is a prerequisite to implementing a program for the patients.

Certainly an essential ingredient in behavior change programs is empirical evaluation of the techniques. To many individuals, evaluation is mistakenly considered as important only when conducting research and may even interfere with treatment. In behavioral programs, the distinction between evaluative research and treatment, even for a single case, is not veridical. Whether treatment is effective is always open to question and is answered with empirical data. It is disconcerting to find programs which are designed to change behavior either of the staff or patients and which fail to evaluate the procedures.

Many of the issues discussed with regard to both staff and patients presuppose that the current institutional structure should be maintained. It is difficult to see how the traditional institutional structure can prepare a patient for outside living in the community. The behaviors developed through individualized or group contingencies can come under the control of the institution unless extrainstitutional life can in some way be integrated. Even when the demands for self-care and individual responsibility are brought into the hospital, complete self-sufficiency is not demanded in the hospital environment. The problem is not a matter of developing behaviors alone, but also the stimulus conditions which come to control those behaviors.

In considering the type of institution best suited to developing effective reinforcement contingencies on a large scale one should be concerned with the type of contingencies and their relation to the patient's release. A setting in which behaviors can be reinforced which are directly relevant to posthospital functioning in many respects is ideal (e.g. Kelley and Hendersen, 1971). Additionally, a setting which approaches identity with the post-hospital setting in which the patient will function is the remaining ideal requirement. The limiting case is a situation in which a patient remains in his extrahospital life completely and his behavior is developed through programs implemented by employers, parents, friends, and himself. An institution which approaches the above requirements would be located directly in the community with patient opportunities for increasingly greater involvement in community activities including employment and socal activities. In such a facility, the stages through which a patient passes can directly involve community placement and follow-up. Reinforcement contingencies can be made to reflect those behaviors required for posthospital adjustment (rather than activity on the ward) under the circumstances in which the patient will function. It will probably be some time before the majority of institutions change in structure. Token programs in hospitals will continue to make advances in effecting behavior change. As these programs proliferate, increasingly greater attention will be devoted to areas related to staff behavior change and patient involvement in their own rehabilitation.

REFERENCES

Axelrod, S.: Comparison of individual and group contingencies in two special classes. *Behav Ther*, 4:83-90, 1973.

Ayllon, T., and Azrin, N. H.: *The Token Economy: A Motivational System for Therapy and Rehabilitation.* New York, Appleton, 1968.

Breyer, N. L., and Allen, G. J.: Effects of Implementing a Token Economy on Teacher Attending Behavior. Paper presented at the Sixth Annual Meeting of the Association for the Advancement of Behavior Therapy, New York, October 1972.

Bricker, W. A.; Morgan, D. G., and Grabowski, J. G.: Development and maintenance of a behavior modification repertoire of cottage attendants through TV feedback. *Am J Ment Defic*, 77:128-136, 1972.

Brown, J.; Montgomery, R., and Barclay, J.: An example of psychologist management of teacher reinforcement procedures in the elementary classroom. *Psychol Sch*, 6:336-340, 1969.

Christopherson, E. R.; Arnold, C. M.; Hill, D. W., and Quilitch, H. R.: The home point system: Token reinforcement procedures for application by parents of children with behavior problems. *J Appl Behav Anal*, 5:485-497, 1972.

Cooper, M. L.; Thomson, C. L., and Baer, D. M.: The experimental modification of teacher attending behavior. *J Appl Behav Anal*, 3:153-157, 1970.

Cossairt, A.; Hall, R. V., and Hopkins, B. L.: The effects of experimenter's instructions, feedback, and praise on teacher praise and student attending behavior. *J Appl Behav Anal*, 6:89-100, 1973.

Fielding, L. T.; Errickson, E., and Bettin, B.: Modification of staff behavior: A brief note. *Behav Ther*, 2:550-553, 1971.

Gardner, J. M.: Teaching behavior modification to nonprofessionals. *J Appl Behav Anal*, 5:517-521, 1972.

Gardner, J. M.: Training the trainers: A review of research on teaching behavior modification. In Rubin, R. D.; Brady, J. P., and Henderson, J. D. (Eds.): *Advances in Behavior Therapy, Volume 4*. New York, Acad Pr, 1973, pp. 145-158.

Hall, J., and Baker, R.: Token economy systems: Breakdown and control. *Behavior Res Ther*, 11:253-263, 1973.

Heap, R. F.; Boblitt, W. E.; Moore, C. H., and Hord, J. E.: Behavior-milieu therapy with chronic neurospychiatric patients. *J Abnorm Psychol*, 76:349-354, 1970.

Katz, R. C.; Johnson, C. A., and Gelfand, S.: Modifying the dispensing of reinforcers: Some implications for behavior modification with hospitalized patients. *Behav Ther*, 3:579-588, 1972.

Kazdin, A. E.: The failure of some patients to respond to token programs. *J Behav Ther Exp Psychiatry*, 4:7-14, 1973a.

Kazdin, A. E.: Methodological and assessment considerations in evaluating reinforcement programs in applied settings. *J Appl Behav Anal*, 6:517-531, 1973b.

Kazdin, A. E.: Recent advances in token economy research. In Hersen, M.; Eisler, R. M., and Miller, P. M. (Eds.): *Progress in Behavior Modification*. New York, Acad Pr, 1975.

Kazdin, A. E.: Self-monitoring and behavior change. In Mahoney, M. J., and Thoresen, C. E. (Eds.): *Self-control: Power to the Person*. Monterey, Brooks-Cole, 1974, pp. 218-246.

Kazdin, A. E., and Bootzin, R. R.: The token economy: An evaluative review. *J Appl Behav Anal*, 5:343-372, 1972.

Kelley, K. M., and Henderson, J. D.: A community-based operant learning environment II: Systems and procedures. In Rubin, R. D.; Fensterheim, H.; Lazarus, A. A., and Franks, C. M. (Eds.): *Advances in Behavior Therapy*. New York, Acad Pr, 1971, pp. 249-250.

Liberman, R.: A view of behavior modification projects in California. *Behav Res Ther*, 6:331-341, 1968.

Lovitt, T. C., and Curtiss, K. A.: Academic response rate as a function of teacher- and self-imposed contingencies. *J Appl Behav Anal*, 2:49-53, 1969.

McReynolds, W. T., and Coleman, J.: Token economy: Patient and staff changes. *Behav Res Ther*, 10:29-34, 1972.

Olson, R. P., and Greenberg, D. J.: Effects of contingency contracting and decision-making groups with chronic mental patients. *J Consult Clin Psychol*, 38:376-383, 1972.

Panyan, M.; Boozer, H., and Morris, N.: Feedback to attendants as a reinforcer for applying operant techniques. *J Appl Behav Anal*, 3:1-4, 1970.

Patterson, R.; Cooke, C., and Liberman, R. P.: Reinforcing the reinforcers: A method of supplying feedback to nursing personnel. *Behav Ther*, 3:444-446, 1972.

Paul, G. L.; McInnis, T. L., and Mariotto, M. J.: Objective performance outcomes associated with two approaches to training mental health technicians in mileu and social-learning programs. *J Abnorm Psychol*, 82:523-532, 1973.

Pomerleau, O. F.; Bobrove, P. H., and Harris, L. C.: Some observations on a controlled social environment for psychiatric patients. *J Behav Ther Exp Psychiatry*, 3:15-21, 1972.

Pomerleau, O. F.; Bobrove, P. H., and Smith, R. H.: Rewarding psychiatric aides for the behavioral improvement of assigned patients. *J Appl Behav Anal*, 6:383-390, 1973.

Redd, W. H.: Effects of mixed reinforcement contingencies on adults' control of children's behavior. *J Appl Behav Anal*, 2:249-254, 1969.

Ringer, V. M. J.: The use of a "token helper" in the management of class-room behavior problems and in teacher training. *J Appl Behav Anal*, 6:671-677, 1973.

Roberts, C. L., and Perry, R. M.: A total token economy. *Ment Retard*, 8:15-18, 1970.

Solomon, R. W., and Wahler, R. G.: Peer reinforcement control of class-room problem behavior. *J Appl Behav Anal*, 6:49-56, 1973.

Suchotliff, L.; Greaves, S.; Stecker, H., and Berke, R.: Critical variables in the token economy. *Proceedings of the 78th Annual Convention of the American Psychological Association*, 5:517-518, 1970.

Ullmann, L. P.: *Institution and Outcome: A Comparative Study of Psychiatric Hospitals*. London, Pergamon, 1967.

Wolf, M. M.; Hanley, E. L.; King, L. A.; Lachowicz, J., and Giles, D. K.: The timer-game: A variable interval contingency for the management of out-of-seat behavior. *Except Child*, 37:113-117, 1970.

Chapter III

TRAINING AND MAINTAINING STAFF BEHAVIORS IN RESIDENTIAL TREATMENT PROGRAMS

Titus McInnis

INTRODUCTION

T HIS CHAPTER CONTAINS a discussion of some of the factors that seem to be important in the initial training and the subsequent maintenance of desirable staff behaviors in residential treatment programs. Attention is also given to the role of organizational variables and the role of structure of treatment programs, both of which appear to underlie successful training and supervisory procedures. Little attention is given to the important subject of selection procedures, and none is given to the influence of institutional administrations or larger political structures which may have strong effects on staff development programs. The focus in this chapter is on in-program administration.

The author's qualifications for writing on these subjects are based on five years experience as program director of a comparative research/treatment project designed to compare social-learning (token system), milieu (therapeutic community), and traditional hospital treatment in the rehabilitation of chronic mental patients.* The author's responsibilities included hiring, training, and general management of paraprofessional and professional staff members. As part of the project a training study was conducted to evaluate the effects of two modes of staff training

---

* Results of the project, which was directed by Gordon L. Paul, will be published in 1975.

on attitudes and performance of paraprofessionals. Reference is made at appropriate places in this chapter to this training study and to other features of this Rehabilitation Project.

References to literature in this chapter focus on those articles most relevant to the treatment situation; however, some attention is given to the management or industrial literature. Information from sources other than treatment applications will be discussed where applicable. While there are many psychological treatment programs which include staff training programs, few reports based on such programs provide information about training and supervision of staff members (Loeber, 1971) or report evaluation of training methods (D'Augelli, 1973; Goldstein and Goedhart, 1973). Our observation is that the literature contains relatively few experimental reports concerned with staff training or maintenance, and that most existing ones were published quite recently. There seems to be a laudable upsurge of interest in the experimental study of staff training and maintenance procedures, probably resulting from a growing realization of the importance of paraprofessionals as change agents.

Our aim in this chapter is to present the reader with specific ideas that he might incorporate into his own treatment setting. The main purpose in citing research is to help restrict the ideas presented to those which have some experimental support. Another aim, with respect to the cited literature, is to present it in such detail that techniques can be applied either unchanged or in adapted form in the reader's situation. Other nonexperimental material is presented, based on the author's or others' experiences, but such anecdotal information is clearly labeled as such.

Nothing in this chapter, whether based on experimentation or experience, should be considered as dogma. The essence, in our opinion, of a good treatment program is continual evaluation and change. Krasner (1970) noted that no treatment procedure should be enshrined. Atthowe (1973) has observed that a good treatment program contains a data collecting system to record resident progress, and so has research elements. One must keep score somehow to assess progress of residents, so that modifications in treatment procedures can be made where indicated. As long as data are being collected, such collection might as well be in the context of an experimental design from which conclusions can be drawn about efficacy of treatment methods. These considerations would seem to apply to staff training and supervision as well as to treatment procedures.

The thesis of this chapter is that the same principles used in the treatment of residents in a treatment program can also be used in the training and supervision of staff members (e.g. Goldstein and Sorcher, 1973). This thesis, while not a novel or uncommon one, is not universally held; some writers suggest that the emphasis be put on selection of staff members who already have the requisite therapeutic skills (e.g. Rappaport, et al., 1973), and others suggest that people cannot be trained in human relationship skills (e.g. Carlaw, 1970). However, the evidence reviewed in this chapter suggests that staff members can be trained to function effectively in even very novel treatment situations (e.g. Paul, et al., 1973; Bricker, et al., 1972). There are also indications from the treatment literature and from the industrial world that measuring work performance and bringing various incentives to bear on good performance has greatly improved employee effectiveness (e.g. Panyan et al., 1970; Fein, 1974).

ORGANIZATIONAL FACTORS

Staff training and the application of consequences to staff members' behavior after initial training are only two aspects of a treatment program. An entire treatment "package" also includes personnel selection procedures, actual treatment techniques, organization of staff functions, internal communication systems, and other organizational factors. Friedlander and Brown (1974) have observed that attempts to change one element of an organization, such as introducing an in-service training program, while ignoring other elements, such as methodology and role relationships, tend to be unsuccessful. While a perfect treatment package cannot be offered to the reader, he should be cautioned to look at the ramifications of any change he makes in his treatment situation. Some of the factors that should be considered are discussed below.

In regard to selection of employees the author can only recommend that if the job requires the ability to read and understand training manuals and the like, some kind of determination should be made whether prospective employees have these abilities. Alternatively, one must be prepared to offer appropriate remediation after employment. It also seems important that applicants have reasonably normal social skills and, in general, be able to serve as good role models for the residents. Some attention should also be paid to the ability of applicants to handle themselves in case of violence. An in-service training program in methods of physically controlling others without hurting them is recommended. The author believes that such training would *decrease* the likelihood of harm to residents or staff members.

Staff incentive programs, in our opinion, must take place in an environment which is itself conducive to good work. Heller (1972) summed up this view quite well: "Place an executive in a well-founded company with whose objectives and style he can identify, and whose growth and drive create personal opportunities and challenge, and where the executive feels secure, appreciated, properly rewarded, and constantly under fair test: There you have the conditions for marvelous motivation." Employees in a treatment program must feel that the program is the very best of its kind and must have a strong commitment to the program's success. Probably the most important influences in fostering these feelings are the actions of the program director and other authorities in the program who must show that they genuinely have the same feelings. If a treatment staff does not have this *esprit de corps*, efforts to employ explicit consequences to influence staff behavior will probably cause more trouble than good.

The risk of alienating staff members by open attempts to control their behavior is a real one. An "aide of the week" award may be viewed by staff members as a "jerk of the week" award. If, though, there is pride in the treatment program and if the program is well designed and generally successful, a fair and nonpunitive incentive system may be included in the program without inciting revolution. There is something to be said for setting precedents with new employees, and if one has the chance to hire all new, "nonchronic" staff members, one has a rare opportunity to matter-of-factly introduce evaluative and incentive procedures at the outset of the program. Then, less resistance to such things as periodic retesting of employees on program principles and procedures should occur.

Even fair evaluation of staff behaviors is likely to be anxiety-provoking and resisted to some degree. Therefore, it is crucial for the program director to have the formal power to evaluate and to apply consequences, positive and negative, based on his evaluation of staff members' behaviors. Our opinion is that the day has come when the scientist-professional truly has a place in the treatment world. The program director should be both in charge of the execution and evaluation (research) of treatment and in charge of all personnel.

The style or manner of presentation of an incentive program is important. If the incentives can be presented as helpful devices to improve the confidence and efficiency of staff members and if they can be presented in such a way that they will be viewed as a kind of game, in which no one is likely to be hurt, then there is a definite advantage.

Friedlander and Brown (1974) commented favorably on the value of such human relationship or organizational factors as sharing of information, solving interpersonal staff problems through discussion of them, participation in decision making, decentralization of authority, job enrichment, etc. While the government of the Rehabilitation Project was definitely not a democracy, an attempt was made to incorporate procedures which would maximize full involvement in the program by all staff members. Traditional professional roles were de-emphasized; however, everyone had a definite set of responsibilities. In any organization a number of tasks or problems will arise that cannot be easily fitted into the available job descriptions. On the Rehabilitation Project such responsibilities would go to the person who showed interest in and ability to handle the situation, and this person could hold any position within the organization.

In other words, the emphasis was on finding the logical person to do a job and not on adherence to official job descriptions. Problems were shared with, and solutions sought from, all employees.

A crucial aspect of an effective program is the control and dissemination of information within it. One type of information is the technical type consisting of new treatment procedures. In addition, there is such information as new personnel policies, other political information, general feedback to staff members, and a multitude of other kinds of information. It is felt that staff morale and effectiveness is enhanced and anxiety lowered when all program information is made available to all employees. On the Rehabilitation Project an attempt was made to meet this goal by means of staff meetings, day-to-day informal contacts, and various written communications. While the author believed that face-to-face communication was best, he found that a few employees always seemed to fail to receive all information in this manner.

To insure that all messages were received by all employees, a memo system was used for both permanent and short-term messages. Permanent messages were those that described procedures that were not likely to be changed in the foreseeable future, e.g. a detailed recording procedure for recording appearance of residents. Short-term messages consisted of announcements (e.g. a description of a new employee) or short-lived procedures (e.g. a special individualized treatment program). Permanent memos were sent to all employees individually, and a memo or policy book, which also included the program treatment manuals, was kept up-to-date and available for use by all employees. All new memos were placed in a special folder. A cover sheet containing the initials of all current employees was attached to each memo. All employees were expected to sign their names by their initials upon reading the memo. The folder was checked weekly, and feedback was given to those employees who had not indicated they had read a memo that had been in the folder for several days. It should be emphasized that this memo system was a supplement to direct verbal communication. The memo system was used to help insure complete dissemination of information and also to help provide a permanent record of policy changes and various events that took place during the project.

On the Rehabilitation Project the only formally scheduled staff meetings were thirty-minute, between-shift reports. These short meetings were found to be quite inadequate. Some of the types of meetings we felt we needed were (1) senior staff meetings, (2) within-shift and between-shift meetings for junior staff, and (3) general all-staff meetings. The functions of these meetings would vary from task-oriented problems solving to working out interpersonal differences among staff members. Meetings of this sort were held but there was always the risk of not having all relevant people present. The purpose of not scheduling these kinds of meetings on a regular basis was to avoid involving people in meaningless bureaucratic activities as opposed to treatment activities. The author believes that it was a mistake not to schedule such meetings and that if such scheduling is done a way can usually be found to maximize attendance by relevant people without causing treatment to suffer. Also, in regard to meetings, the author has several suggestions: (1) Schedule meetings to last at least one and a half hours; (2) have the meetings regularly even if some of them do not seem necessary; (3) for problem solving meetings, appoint someone to solicit items for, and to distribute, an agenda, and to write and distribute minutes; (4) for meetings devoted to solving interpersonal problems, restrict personal feedback to behavior and forbid attacks on character.

Even if all organizational aspects of the treatment program are very good, no treatment program will be without rough spots in its operation. It is likely that a *very* smoothly running treatment program will not be an effective one. Glaser and Taylor (1973) examined characteristics of successful vs. unsuccessful applied research projects and found that unsuccessful projects tended to be characterized by calm and uneventful interactions among staff members, while successful projects tended to be characterized by stormy, and even heated, interactions among staff members as they worked out the issues relating to the design and implementation of the program. Directors of unsuccessful projects tended to discourage suggestions and criticisms from staff members, to restrict information to a staff elite, and not to share problems with staff members. Directors of successful projects tended to search for advice and criticism, maximize both formal and informal communication, and share project problems with all staff members.

IMPORTANCE OF STRUCTURE

The degree of structure or specification of procedures may be crucial to the success of a treatment program and to training and staff supervision programs. The importance of job analysis and specification has been stressed by Distefano and Pryer (1973) and by Ayllon and Azrin (1968). A treatment program may have all the desirable organizational features discussed above, but fail from lack of clear direction of staff efforts. Detailed specification of programmatic procedures greatly facilitates the training of staff members. Treatment manuals, recording forms, and treatment protocols become the lesson plans not only for didactic instruction, including role playing, but also for on-the-job training and supervision. In addition, such specification facilitates success of the treatment program itself, partly by helping to bring specific, well thought out, or experimentally supported procedures into the treatment effort and partly by allowing for detailed evaluation of therapeutic procedures.

Some of the above points were well illustrated by a case study presented by Smith and Carlin (1972). The study suggested that increased specification of treatment procedures facilitated improvement in staff actions, staff attitudes, and resident behavior. In a short-term treatment ward, a young female resident showing delusions, postural mannerisms, screaming, crying, tantrums, and other distressing behaviors including demands for drugs was admitted. The first attempt at treatment was to give her various drugs and daily psychotherapy sessions. None of this improved her behavior, and she increased her demand for drugs. The next treatment procedure was to start a behavior modification program. The latter program consisted of general instructions to staff members to ignore the resident's "crazy" behaviors, to send her to her room if she persisted in disturbing others, and to pay attention to her when she behaved appropriately. Weekend passes were made contingent on a week of appropriate behavior. Dosage of drugs was to be eliminated, except apparently on an "as needed" basis, on the ground that giving her drugs on demand merely reinforced her demand for them. All these apparently good procedures resulted in increases in her violence and even more demands for drugs. Staff members began to complain that the resident was "really psychotic" and should not be punished. Other staff members went beyond the "time out in room" procedure, and instead, would tie the resident down in her bed for several hours at a time. Staff members began to insist that they could not control the resident's behavior without use of drugs, even though the records of her drug needs indicated that the resident was actually receiving more drugs than before the behavior modification program started. The nurses began to quarrel with the doctors over these issues. Finally, another treatment plan was instituted. This time, a point system was introduced which detailed the behaviors which would earn points for the resident and the misbehaviors which would cost the resident points. Reinforcement was contingent upon specific numbers of points accumulated by the resident. Interestingly, one of the back-up reinforcers used was drugs, though the system was set up so that it was more to the resident's advantage to spend her points for passes than for drugs. After two days of continued difficult behavior, improvement in the resident was noticed. Within one and a half weeks her outbursts ceased, her postural mannerisms were much reduced, and she had taken several successful passes (which were contingent on earning points). She was then discharged without drugs, and she herself commented that the point system had helped her. Of more importance here, the staff members changed their minds about the behavior modification program and later suggested it be tried with other residents. The authors interpreted the improvement in staff attitudes and behavior as resulting from the increased structuring of the treatment program, noting that failure of the first behavior modification program was probably partly due to depriving the nurses of a high frequency behavior, drug disbursement, without giving them a substitute behavior. The second, more structured program gave the nurses another activity, point disbursement, which helped give them the feeling that they were doing something in the name of treatment.

In the above case study the second behavior modification program included recording forms and procedures for keeping track of points earned and lost by the resident. It is very possible that such mechanical aspects of a treatment program themselves control staff behaviors. This control comes from the feedback inherent in precisely detailed work. Feedback may constitute a reinforcer, but it also provides for an immediate focusing of staff attention on behavior required of them. An analogy may be made to the airplane pilot's situation. His motivation to fly and land the plane successfully can be assumed. No "pilot of the week" or other reward would seem necessary to motivate him. The pilot's performance is fed back to him in many ways, including his observation of the many dials which report the airplane's situation. The feedback is immediate and precise, and the pilot makes corrections in his behavior as indicated by the information. In the treatment situation, specification facilitates precise feedback and aids the employee in judging the quality of his own work. Consequences may be attached to specific performances, but there is nothing in the nature of feedback, as such, that implies the application of consequences.

While the tenor of this chapter, to this point, suggests that the author would definitely recommend the use of such procedures as point systems with staff members, such is not the case. If a treatment program is carefully specified, if the employees are enthusiastic about doing a good job, and if praise and censure seem to be motivating to the employees, then the application of consequences other than social ones may not be necessary. In fact, the addition of tangible reinforcers to a well functioning social reinforcement procedure may backfire. In this author's opinion, all that may be needed is a plan which insures that the necessary feedback and subsequent social reinforcement is, in fact, given.

Several aspects of the Rehabilitation Project can serve as examples of the kind of specification under discussion here.

Detailed work schedules for employees were written for two treatment units for three shifts. Each shift alternated work on the two different treatment units, with the day shift making the unit change at noon daily, and evening and night shifts making the change at the start of each full work day. Thus, each staff member learned the schedule of activities and the detailed procedures appropriate to both experimental treatment units. The schedules included the times activities should start, which employee announced the activity, which employee recorded attendance (when such recording was appropriate), which employee had supporting duties, which recording forms were to be used, and when the activity was to cease. All employees were assigned a different number for every day they worked, and the numbers cued the day's duties for them. For example, on a particular day an employee might be Change Agent 1. When he came to work he would note his number for the day, consult the schedule, and then would know what his duties that day would be. Change Agent 2 would also have specified duties, etc. Overall, it was stressed that there really were jobs that had to be performed and that pitching in to help with them all was expected, even if a person were not formally scheduled to perform them. The latter expectation was promulgated to take care of the many unforeseen events that can take place during a treatment day. It can easily be seen that supervision was facilitated by this scheduling system. As Ayllon and Azrin (1968) pointed out, once the staff schedule is set, the supervisor knows where and when to go to observe specific activities and specific staff members.

Recording forms on the Rehabilitation Project served several functions, including, of course, recording of resident progress in many areas. In addition, they served as discriminative stimuli for staff behavior. Colman and Boren (1969) noted that records of resident behavior can serve as implicit instructions to staff members. The recording forms on the Rehabilitation Project provided both implicit and explicit instructions to guide staff behavior. For example, the form used to record meal behavior contained a list of nine criteria deemed to constitute good table manners, e.g. proper use of utensils, so that staff members could be reminded of the criteria as they made their recordings. The entire meal procedure, of which behavior recording was just a part, was taught to staff members from a manual written for this purpose. Among other things, more detailed specification of the meaning of the nine meal behavior criteria was presented in the manual. The meal behavior form listed the names of the current residents in the treatment program and contained column headings for breakfast, lunch, and dinner. On the form used in the social-learning program (the token system) space was also provided for recording tokens disbursed and whether the token was a shaping token (given when the resident improved his performance over the previous meal but still did not meet the highest criterion), or a terminal token (given when the performance met the highest criterion). Treatment manuals specified the kinds of verbalizations to be made by staff members upon delivery or nondelivery of tokens, and the spaces on the form for recording token disbursement served as signals that these verbalizations were to be made. Thus, this meal behavior form contained a wealth of cues which helped to govern staff behavior.

By means of schedules, recording forms, and of even more importance, detailed treatment protocols based on task analyses, staff members' behaviors can be specified in such a way as to facilitate staff training, maintenance of staff behaviors, resident improvement, and evaluation of treatment procedures. In an earlier section of this chapter we stressed that treatment programs should also be experimental programs. A treatment program that is always being evaluated for effectiveness will be a dynamic and probably successful one. The question arises as to how a periodically examined and changed program can also be one that embodies the careful and relentless specification recommended above. How can one be rigid and flexible at the same time? We think the answer lies in making aspects of the treatment program rigid for short periods of time. Rigidity, in this case, is not a bad thing. It is, in fact, a necessary condition for any evaluation of procedures. One must try out a specified procedure without any modifications for a period of time if one is to test its effectiveness. While certain kinds of flexibility are always desirable, e.g. the judgment to give or hold back a reinforcer, such flexibility should still fall with a set of guiding rules.

Change in a treatment program should always follow an adequate tryout of a treatment procedure and evaluation of its effectiveness. Flexibility should be the rule after, but not during, time-limited treatment procedures.

STAFF TRAINING

This section is devoted to training methods for paraprofessionals and includes presentations of several specific model training programs that the author thinks have merit. The emphasis here is not on content of training programs, but rather on teaching methods. One of the issues in training is whether formal academic training in treatment philosophies or principles is more or less important than on-the-job training. The trend, as will be seen, is toward on-the-job training, but the issue has certainly not been settled. There does seem to be agreement, though, that on-the-job training is absolutely essential. All the training programs presented here were conducted by professionals directly involved in treatment situations. In no case was training conducted by a centralized training division within an institution. As a general recommendation we can state flatly that one must design and conduct one's own training program in one's own treatment situation. One cannot rely on training conducted by people not intimately associated with and involved in the actual treatment program for which people are being trained.

The Academic vs. On-the-job Training Issue

Gardner (1972) began training in behavior modification with one group of attendants by assigning them to six one-hour role-playing sessions wherein the attendants worked in pairs, assuming roles of resident trainers and residents alternately, all under the supervision of a staff trainer who provided a role model. Another group of attendants were simultaneously entered into a lecture series of eight one-hour classes on behavior modification principles. After each group had completed its respective initial training, it received the other mode of training. A test of knowledge of behavior modification principles, given after the initial training of both groups was completed, showed superiority for the group that had had the classroom training. A test of proficiency in applying behavior modification skills, given at the same time, showed superiority for the group that was offered the role-playing mode of training. After both groups had received both modes of training, there were no differences between the groups on either of the dependent measures. The author concluded that principles may be best taught by lecture, while actual proficiency in applying techniques may be best taught by a method which emphasizes performance skills.

Cone and Sheldon (1973) noted that training in principles has not generally led to relevant on-the-job performance in the past and that a movement to more practical training seems to be under way. In their training study, nine recently employed aides were taught eight behaviors including three antecedent behaviors (verbal prompts, physical prompts, and modeling) and five consequent behaviors (general verbal praise, specific verbal praise, physical reinforcement, material reinforcement, and time out). The first training procedure involved showing the trainees a thirty-minute videotape which defined and gave examples of the eight desired behaviors. The latter procedure constituted a kind of academic presentation of material. This training procedure resulted in a small decrease in overall percentage of antecedent behaviors and a small increase in overall percentage of consequent behaviors. The second training procedure consisted of remote auditory prompting presented by a professional staff member from a wireless FM microphone to a radio and then to earphones worn by the trainees. An example of a physical prompt was, "Raise his arm." This prompting procedure produced large increases in both antecedent and consequent behaviors. The authors did not conclude that on-the-job training was superior to academic training in spite of their results. Application of consequences was increased by the videotape film, and one consequence in particular, general verbal praise, increased in this condition to a level almost the same as that achieved during the prompting condition. The authors did conclude that both didactic and on-the-job training was probably needed and that the task of the experimenter should be to determine which behaviors are most amenable to which method. Given the necessary equipment, the reader probably could use videotape and auditory prompting to good advantage, as did these authors. The reader should also note the great specificity of target behaviors employed in the investigation. This specification allowed results to emerge that could not have if the usual global staff ratings had been used.

Paul, et al. (1973) and Paul and McInnis (1974) reported studies of the effects of different methods of training on attitudes and performance of paraprofessionals in the Rehabilitation Project. One trainee group received all training prior to arrival of residents at the treatment site and prior to institution of treatment programs—the training consisting of classroom reading of treatment manuals, lectures, large and small group discussions, films, and role playing, all conducted by professional staff members. The second group of trainees received the same content as the first group, but training by professionals was augmented by trainee assignment to experienced technicians who demonstrated procedures with actual residents and discussed them with the trainees. At the completion of the initial training phase and upon assignment of trainees to their work shifts, further on-the-job training was provided, the first group receiving it from professional staff members and the latter group receiving it from experienced technicians. An employee who was entering the on-shift phase of his training received a training form which contained a list of all the major duties required of employees on his particular shift and spaces for recording date, observations, and "carry out with instructions." For each specific duty the trainee was initially expected to observe an experienced technician perform it at least three times. Then the trainee was expected to attempt the task under supervision at least eight times. A final checkout for each duty was performed by a professional staff member. Assessment of knowledge by a test of material covered during the training prior to shift assignment showed superiority for the group that received all training by professionals prior to the initiation of the treatment programs. Assessment of on-the-job performance, employing research observers who observed staff-resident interactions on an average ten-minute-on/ten-minute-off schedule during all waking hours of the residents, showed superiority for the group that had training by experienced employees in the actual treatment situation. The authors did not conclude that academic training was valueless, since knowledge of principles was found to be positively correlated with good on-the-job performance in both trainee groups. For a detailed description of the content of the training program the reader is directed to Paul and McInnis (1974).

Final conclusions cannot be drawn as yet on the issue of on-the-job vs. academic training. The data presented above, however, seem to support on-the-job training over academic instruction in the production of good on-the-job performance. One could summarize the data by saying simply: "One gets what one trains." However, the study by Cone and Sheldon (1973) suggested that academic training can have beneficial effects on some aspects of performance.

The literature cited above suggests that classroom instruction is relatively less effective than on-the-job instruction in training most good job performances. However, the present author clings to the view that it is important that staff members understand why they do what they do, so that in the actual treatment situation rational decisions can be made when things do not go smoothly and according to plan. On the Rehabilitation Project there were one or two employees who tended to follow the rules to the letter under all circumstances. Needless to say, these employees were sometimes a source of satisfaction and sometimes a source of great frustration to us. We believe that the answer may lie in teaching treatment principles *in vivo* along with the procedures in a variety of situations so that each trainee becomes capable of self-generation of procedures in novel situations.

Model Training Programs

Goldstein and Goedhart (1973) reported two experiments designed to increase empathic behaviors in psychiatric nurses. Previous research by Goldstein, et al. (1971) had shown that simple exposure to a model for about one hour could increase a behavior deemed to be therapeutic, but that the effect did not transfer, even one hour later, to an *in vivo* test of the new skill. The new studies, in which groups of six to eight students were trained, were designed to increase the staying power of the training. The "structured learning" training procedures employed in the first study constituted what was intended to be a model training program, the chief characteristic of which, in the author's opinion, was its thoroughness.

The training included (1) a verbal presentation of the meaning and importance of empathy, (2) presentation of a scale which concretely illustrated empathic behaviors, (3) discussion of related issues, e.g. empathy vs. sympathy, (4) modeling of thirty simulated staff-resident interactions in which empathy was demonstrated by two instructors, one of whom acted as the nurse and one as the resident, with instructions to trainees to silently role play what would have been their own responses if they had been playing the roles, (5) role playing by trainees wherein simulated resident statements were read aloud by a trainer who then asked for volunteers to respond empathically (then called on trainees in turn), (6) repeating the role playing sequence twice so that each trainee could respond to several "resident" statements and be praised for empathic responses, (7) one or two similar but extended role-playing sessions in which trainees responded both to standard situations and situations suggested by trainees, and (8) a final demonstration by the two trainers of the standard situations and how to respond to them empathically. This training took a total of ten hours spread over two days. As compared with an untrained control group, trainees who received the above training not only showed increased ability to make empathic responses, but also maintained the ability on a follow-up test given one month later. The second experiment was a repetition of the first one with the addition of a group that, in addition to the ten hours of "structured learning" training received two week of on-the-job supervision and training by two trainers who also provided daily fifteen-minute sessions during which verbatim records of actual interactions with residents were discussed and evaluated. During the latter sessions the trainer offered feedback and further modeling of the desired empathic responses. Results of this second experiment replicated the first one and also indicated that the *in vivo* training enhanced the transfer of training to the on-the-job situation. These studies illustrated the use of verbal instruction, modeling, role playing, and on-the-job supervision as effective training methods. The second study also offers support to the idea that on-the-job training can add something to even the most thorough academic training. Very thorough training, especially "round robin" role playing as illustrated in these studies, can be very boring to everyone concerned, but there seems to be no substitute for making sure that every trainee gets a chance to respond to at least several representative stimulus situations. Similar thoroughness in training all targeted staff behaviors useful in token economies would take much time, but again, there does not seem to be an easy way out of the necessity to be thorough.

Martin, et al. (1973), after noting that academic training has not seemed to have much effect on on-the-job behavior of nursing trainees, described a procedure designed to train work behaviors of nurses. This procedure is quite similar to the one reported by Paul and McInnis (1974). The procedure described by Martin, et al. (1973) included (1) presentation of all written procedures and data sheets for each activity, (2) an explanation of each activity by a regular staff member, (3) observation of each activity, with the demonstrator of each activity being required to ask the trainees three questions to test their understanding of the procedure, (4) actual tryout of procedures by the trainee, sometimes with the demonstrator carrying out the first part of the procedure, (5) trainee conducting an entire therapy session to the satisfaction of the instructor, (6) trainee conducting therapy without supervision, and (7) a final written examination on general ward procedures and data sheets. This on-the-job training procedure was recorded on a form listing activities on the left side and the various instructional procedures across the top, so that notations could be made in the body of the form of the progress of each trainee in learning each activity. The authors noted, however, that even with these training procedures, it was necessary to reinforce staff members for continued good work performance. Their suggestions of how to do this are reported below in the section on maintenance of staff behaviors.

Watson, et al. (1971) describe a very thorough training

program (see Chapter IV in this book). This program included both classroom and on-the-job training. An interesting feature of the training program was a series of academic and behavioral tests that had to be passed at the 90-percent level before the students could progress through the program.

The training programs summarized above illustrate a number of training procedures that may be adapted by the reader. None of these procedures were particularly novel or original ones; however, they were all quite thorough. It is perhaps true that the characteristic that best discriminates successful from unsuccessful training (or treatment) programs is not the application of new and brilliant ideas, but rather the unwavering application of fundamental principles.

Atthowe (1973) has noted that initial success of a treatment program can sometimes result in complacency and cessation of efforts to reinforce staff members. Martin, et al. (1973) observed that even after careful and successful initial training, programmatic staff behaviors must still be reinforced. So, a discussion of several procedures that have been used to maintain good staff behavior follows.

MAINTAINING STAFF BEHAVIORS

A variety of incentives have been used to maintain staff behaviors in treatment programs, with some programs employing several incentives in the same program. Surprisingly, there are a fair number of articles reporting the use of money (or trading stamps) as reinforcers for staff members. An early, but non-experimental, report of this nature was presented by Wolf, et al. (1968) who gave a ten-dollar award every six weeks to instructors whose students' grade point average improved. Aside from money, other incentives that have been frequently reported include praise, censure, public recognition, group pressure, simple supervision, monitoring of staff behaviors by research observers or by the residents themselves, and feedback of resident or employee performance. Reports concerned with the latter types of incentives are presented below under the (slightly inaccurate) heading, "Feedback and Social Reinforcement." The reports concerned with monetary or similar incentives are grouped under the heading, "Money as an Incentive."

Feedback and Social Reinforcement

Colman and Boren (1969) found that a point matrix, which showed points earned by residents for targeted behaviors, served as a set of instructions to staff members by indicating action to be taken based on current functioning of residents as indicated by the record of point earnings and spendings. The point matrices were monitored both by staff members and by residents, and the residents tended to insure that the point system was administered fairly by staff members. The authors also reported an example of how a record system can cue unwanted staff behaviors. An early form of the data matrix highlighted residents who were spending more points than they earned, that is, functioning poorly within the system. The latter record directed the attention of staff members to poorly functioning residents more than to better functioning residents. The data form was therefore redesigned to eliminate negative balances, fines were assessed once a week (by vote of staff and residents), and debts were paid off not with points but with extra work. The effect of the change in the form was to direct staff members' attention to numbers of points earned, rather than to points lost.

A resident of the week was chosen by staff members in the above program basing the choice on data in the point matrices. Having to choose well functioning residents on this weekly basis and for longer intervals tended to force staff members to review records on a regular basis. This procedure also served to focus staff members' attention on positive improvement of residents. While the record system itself tended to support and maintain programmatic staff behaviors, the authors had to use directed review of certain behavioral indices during two weekly staff meetings along with social reinforcement (praise) when appropriate. The behavioral indices used for this purpose depicted general results of the treatment program and were not individual records of residents, over which the residents themselves had some control.

The above report highlights the use of record systems, as such, to control staff members' behaviors, and it adds the intriguing use of residents' monitoring of their own records as a means of motivating staff members to properly conduct the treatment program. Even more extensive use of resident involvement has been explored by Phillips, et al. (1973) who examined the possibility of bringing residents into the administration of the treatment program itself.

Panyan, et al. (1970) provided staff members with a feedback sheet listing the total possible number of training sessions they could conduct (with residents) and the total actually conducted by them and found large increases in percent of sessions conducted. The feedback sheet contained the names and percentage of sessions conducted for all staff members on the treatment unit, and in addition the performance records of other treatment units were publicly posted. Here the operating variables seemed to have been not only feedback, as such, but also competition within the treatment unit and competition with other units.

Barton, et al. (1970) trained attendants to apply contingencies to meal behaviors of retarded residents. Training of staff members was by means of verbal instructions and modeling, and maintenance of staff members' behaviors was facilitated by public posting of the daily contingencies for the residents, by research observers checking on staff performance, and by showing the staff members graphs of resident progress. Which type of staff control was best was not evaluated. The authors speculated that the most important influences on staff members' behavior were the obvious improvement of the residents and the feeling of staff members that they had control over the residents' behavior.

Patterson, et al. (1972) published a weekly newsletter for staff members in a behavior modification program, one feature of which was the publication of noteworthy achievements by staff members. (See Chapter V in this book.)

Cossairt, et al. (1973) attempted to get teachers to praise their students and compared the effects of instructions, feedback, and praise on this behavior. The authors found inconclusive results with instructions alone and with a combination of instructions and feedback, but did find that adding praise to the other two procedures resulted in significant increases in teacher praise.

Favell (1973) increased punctual behavior in a group of professional staff members. The setting was a regular staff meeting, and the intervention was giving feedback to each staff member during meetings about his lateness record. Each person who came to the meeting was shown a sheet which showed him how late he was for the present meeting and his record for previous meetings. The data sheet also contained similar data for all others who were scheduled to attend the meeting—thus an element of competition was present in the procedure. The author did not tie any consequences to staff members' lateness, and indeed, reported some hesitation about doing so on the grounds that such action might have damaged his professional relationships with the other members of the group. In fact, though, the feedback procedure as presented was accepted good-naturedly by the group members.

Watson, et al. (1971) reported the use of several incentives for staff members in an institution for the mentally retarded. These incentives included time off from work, increased authority to make changes in the treatment program, and the placing of photos of outstanding staff members on a "Recognition Bulletin Board." (See Chapter IV.)

On the Rehabilitation Project efforts to maintain staff members' programmatic behaviors were mainly restricted to the use of social reinforcement. However, more substantial back-up reinforcers were available, including on the positive side, raises, promotions, assignment to a desired shift, and letters of commendation; and on the negative side, failure to give raises, demotions, letters of reprimand, suspension without pay, and actual dismissal. Much time was spent in the development of feedback systems which insured that each employee would be continually aware of the quality of his performance and his standing in relation to his job security. As much delivery of positive and negative feedback as was feasible was encouraged, so that a verbally reinforcing milieu became the norm. Gossip and backbiting were discouraged by not allowing anyone to criticize anyone else unless the other person was present to hear the criticism, and by arranging staff meetings for the purpose of interpersonal feedback. Several formal information gathering and feedback systems were instituted. Information about staff behaviors came from several sources. Any staff member could turn in an "Excellence Report" on any other staff member. There was also a "Staff Supervision and Program Troubleshooting Form" for use by supervisors. Programmatic errors and excellent performances were reported by research observers on appropriate forms. Errors on recording sheets were noted by clerical personnel and reported on a "Recording Error Form."

All of these reports were presented personally to the individual employee by a professional staff member soon after they were written. Feedback based on the reports was given in an emotionally neutral and nonpunitive manner (except that praise was given enthusiastically), and if a report was questioned, the employee and the writer of the report were brought together to discuss it.

Periodically it was necessary to rate each employee on a state personnel rating form. For established employees, this rating was required once a year. New employees received ratings at intervals during their first year of employment. An effort was made to make these state ratings meaningful. Vague criteria for job performance printed on the state form were translated into more specific criteria relating to the actual jobs of employees. In addition to the required ratings, each employee received unofficial three-month and six-month ratings prior to the yearly required rating. All reports of staff behavior from any source, and records of absenteeism and tardiness were used as bases for these evaluations. In addition, peer ratings were solicited prior to each formal evaluation. These ratings were shown to the rated employees, so that no secrecy was involved. A rating was summarized in a feedback letter from the program director which contained all available information plus his comments. The comments would sometimes include suggestions about behaviors which should be changed and a clear statement of consequences (positive and negative) if the behavior did not change in a reasonable time. This feedback system kept the employees informed about their status and provided periodic summaries of their job performance. Above all, the three-month, six-month, one-year schedule gave the employee time to modify his behavior before any drastic action was taken. It was a slow and a fair system about which we had few complaints—even from those few people who did suffer serious negative consequences.

A frequent problem in any treatment program is absenteeism or lateness. On the Rehabilitation Project we attacked the lateness problem by having a secretary note the time of arrival of employees. The information was given to the program director who disseminated a monthly record sheet showing the lateness record of all employees. Though we did not test this procedure experimentally, the data did show less lateness after the feedback system started. Absenteeism can be an even more serious problem. In the Illinois system, a sick day was awarded by the state every month to every employee, and unused days accumulated indefinitely. There was no reward, such as payment upon leaving state service, for sick days not taken. Since we deliberately employed a minimum number of employees to run our programs on a day-to-day basis, the absence of an employee for any reason was disturbing to everyone, especially to fellow employees who had to take on the duties of the missing employee. In addition, the nature of the programs themselves dictated that a minimum number of employees be present. One problem for an administrator is how to tell true from faked sickness, especially when the employee simply calls in sick. Our answer to that problem was to not try to make that determination. Excessive absenteeism, for any reason, tended to lower staff evaluations, unless there were very clear extenuating circumstances. The heart of the control system we eventually set up was a monthly report showing the number of sick days an employee had taken since his entry into state service divided by the total number he could have accumulated if he had never taken a sick day. The higher the percentage, the worse was the record. The report was broken down by shift for the technician-level personnel and by functional groups, e.g. educational staff, for other staff members, so that competition could develop among staff groups. Use of sick days did decline after this system was instituted, and there were some clear indications that chronic users of sick days, who were fairly obviously using them for purposes other than sickness, received pressures from fellow staff members to cease that practice.

Money as an Incentive

Because a study by Loeber (1971) was a laboratory experiment not involving actual residents, it will not be presented in detail here. Loeber, however, concluded that staff behavior improved more when it was rewarded with money than when it was rewarded by resident improvement.

An experiment by Bricker, et al. (1972) may be more of a training study than a staff maintenance study; however, the distinction between training and maintenance is not a clear one and the staff members studied in the experiment were already working employees at the outset of the experiment. The report of the study did not indicate that the staff members had received a formal training program, though they had been active in the Neighborhood Youth Corps, sponsored by the U.S. Office of Economic Opportunity. They had also successfully demonstrated the capability to work effectively with mentally retarded children if under direct and continuous supervision. There were nine staff members in the experiment who trained five retarded children in various skills. The dependent variables in the investigation were the amount of time the staff members spent "on task" and the suitability of content of the training sessions for the children, the staff members being free to choose the content. A two-week baseline period during which videotaped samples of the staff members' work performance were taken revealed that the staff members spent most of their time talking with each other in a kitchen or in reading magazines. In addition, during the baseline period, the suitability of content of the resident training was essentially nil. After the baseline period, the staff members were assembled and shown videotapes of their just previous training performance. Feedback on the quality of selection of training materials and on the quality of the interactions with the children was also given to the staff members. Trading stamps, costing an average of fifteen cents per staff member per training session, were given to the staff members for high-quality staff-resident interactions, as shown on the videotape, and also were given for the amount of time each trainee spent on a task, at the rate of one stamp for each minute. The result of this procedure was a dramatic increase in the amount of time the trainees spent with the children. The investigation included other manipulations, but just one of them will be mentioned here. A subgroup of four staff members was identified which accounted for most of the failures in the staff group to show good-quality interactions with the children. Individuals in this subgroup were given additional training focused on a reduction in the frequency of punishment, an increase in the amount of prompting and fading, and better use of reinforcement. These staff members received an extra half-hour of instruction daily which involved making a ten-minute videotape of each staff member's performance that day as he interacted with a child and subsequent discussion of the staff member's performance as shown on the videotape of the ten-minute session. A point system was used which enabled each of the staff members to earn as many as fifty trading stamps for his performance during the ten-minute session. These procedures improved the performance of these four staff members on each of the targeted behaviors, with only the fading of prompts showing no more than modest improvement. The authors reported that their training procedures resulted in a 700-percent increase in the amount of interaction between staff members and the children and that the percentage of time that each child was engaged in a task of value to him increased from zero to 71 percent by the end of the eight-week study. No data was presented on the progress of the children themselves. In this study the presence of a TV monitor in the classroom at all times, plus the knowledge by staff members that it might be recording their behaviors at any time, probably served as a means of continual supervision, but one that, in fact, only periodically required actual intervention by supervisors. The addition of detailed feedback and the reward of trading stamps served to increase not only on-task behavior itself but also specific classes of behaviors thought to be therapeutic for the children.

Katz, et al. (1972) studied the effects of instructions, prompts, and monetary rewards on the content of interactions between aides and residents. Specific resident behaviors were categorized as "task-oriented" or "inappropriate." Aide behaviors were categorized as "positive interaction," "negative interaction," or "neutral interaction." During a baseline condition, in which staff-resident interactions were systematically observed and recorded, interactions of *any* kind were rare, even though one of the three residents studied often exhibited reinforceable behaviors. The aides were then told to administer positive consequences, such as praise and cigarettes, to the residents when they were task-oriented. These instructions had little effect on the aides' behavior. The next step was to have an "undergraduate" remind or prompt the aides in the actual treatment situation to deliver the positive consequences. The latter procedure resulted in a slight increase in number of reinforcements delivered by the aides, and in the two poorly performing residents an increase in task-oriented behavior. After the prompting phase of the study, four of the aides were told that they would receive fifteen dollars if the frequency of which task-oriented behavior was reinforced by the aides rose to approximately 50 percent of the observations of staff-resident interactions—for two consecutive days. The monetary award produced an increase in percentage of positive interactions from 8 percent in the prompt condition to 70 percent in the monetary award condition. A follow-up period, which lacked promise of money, showed a decrease to 23 percent of positive interactions. Data on task orientation of the residents showed parallel increases and decreases. In this experiment the use of a student prompter was probably not very powerful as compared to the use of a professional prompter (cf. Cone and Sheldon, 1973). These authors are to be commended for reporting resident as well as staff data, and it is interesting that what was rewarded with the money was the combination of good resident performance and good staff performance.

Though their data were not gathered in a treatment situation, a study designed to increase punctuality in industrial workers by Hermann, et al. (1973) is relevant to the present discussion. These authors made daily payments to employees in an industrial firm in Mexico of slips of paper redeemable for two pesos (16¢

in U.S. currency). A maximum of ten pesos (80¢ in U.S. currency) could be obtained by each employee when he turned in his accumulated tokens at the end of the week. This bonus money was paid in addition to the weekly pay of these employees, which was fifty pesos ($4 in U.S. currency). The bonus system was superimposed on an incentive system already in use in the factory which involved annual money awards to workers with the best attendance and punctuality records. In addition, the factory had a long-standing policy of suspending workers for one day without salary if they were tardy three times within thirty days. The new bonus pay system resulted in increases in punctuality for an experimental group as compared to a control group which was not given the bonus money. The authors noted that their bonus procedure might not be considered a practical one because of the paperwork involved, but suggested that it might be used as a remedial procedure and then gradually stretched out from a daily bonus to a monthly or bimonthly bonus. A practical problem, of course, is how to get the money for such a reward system. Large amounts of money might be needed. For example, the weekly eighty-cent bonus mentioned about represented 20 percent of the average weekly salaries of the factory employees—the equivalent of an average day's pay.

Martin, et al. (1973) presented two studies. In the first, nurses, aides, and attendants in an institution for the mentally retarded were offered a chance to participate in a staff incentive program. Programmatic staff behaviors would be rewarded with points redeemable in backup reinforcers such as a half-hour talk with the supervisor, a free beer at a pub with the supervisor, opportunity to work with a favorite resident, or opportunity to not work with the residents for a day or so. This plan was rejected by the staff members, but later accepted when thirty-eight dollars per three-week shift was offered as an additional backup, with the staff member earning the most points receiving twenty dollars, the next ten dollars, and the next eight dollars. Staff behaviors that were reinforced included completing training sessions and taking on extra training sessions with residents. Results of this study included a more than double increase in the percent of individual resident training sessions conducted. However, improvement of residents was very minimal. This lack of significant improvement of residents was explained by noting that the actual training programs, while carried out well, were poorly designed for the residents to which they were applied. Individual staff members had been given the freedom to design the individual programs. Not only did the residents not improve significantly, but side effects of the staff incentive program were increased staff complaints and even disruption of the treatment program. In the second study a maximum of thirty-eight dollars was offered to staff members every three weeks, but the money was paid contingent on improvement of the residents at the rate of fifty cents per resident behavior trained. This procedure did not increase the number of resident training sessions conducted by the staff members, but it did result in an improvement in resident behavior, followed by a decrease during a return to baseline wherein no monetary awards were given to the staff.

The results of the two experiments indicated that reinforcement of staff members for improvement of residents in their charge did result in improvement of residents, while reinforcement of staff members for conforming to a list of specified staff behaviors thought to be therapeutic did not result in improvement of residents. The staff group in the second study, whose behavior was not directly monitored and used as a basis for the monetary awards, did not gripe about being under surveillance or about the incentive system in general, and in addition, showed several positive behaviors, including a tendency to focus attention on the behavior of the residents, to show concern about resident improvement, to insure that competent staff members performed all training sessions with their residents, to try a variety of reinforcers instead of relying on a last minute search for whatever reinforcers were available, and to pay close attention to summary data indicating their residents' performance.

Pomerleau, et al. (1973) presented data which suggested that monetary awards to staff members contingent on resident improvement increased resident improvement. An aide of the week was chosen on the basis of improvement of two residents assigned to each aide, with the chosen person receiving a weekly cash award. As the monetary awards increased in successive weeks from ten to twenty to thirty dollars, behavior of all residents in the treatment program improved correspondingly. In addition to the above awards, there was a weekly twenty-dollar-award for the most cooperative aide, who was chosen by secret ballot by the aides themselves. The purpose of the latter award was to control the effect of noncontingent awards and to prevent staff disruption due to competition for the other awards. For experimental reasons there was a planned reduction in the amount of the regular award after the gains mentioned above, from thirty to twenty dollars, which resulted in a marked decrease in the quality of resident behavior, complaints from the aides, and threats by the aides to do less work.

The final condition in the experiment produced the worst resident performance. This last condition apparently was the result of a purge within the institution which resulted in cessation of requirements to maintain the token economy and the elimination of psychologists as supervisors of the treatment program. Even though the program was at an end, except for collection of data on resident performance, the remaining aide-level staff members "decided among themselves to continue the transactions of the token economy and to resist pressure from the new clinical director to resume custodial duties" (Pomerleau, et al., 1973, p. 389). The top monetary award in this study, thirty dollars, amounted to a day's pay for these employees, but in this case it was awarded to only one employee weekly. Such a competition for monetary awards might be more affordable than a system wherein every employee stands to receive the award.

Pommer and Streedbeck (1974) employed two procedures to improve job performance of child-care workers. One procedure involved posting of itemized lists of jobs expected of each worker. The other procedure consisted of paying the workers job slips redeemable at the end of each month for one dollar for every job completed. Results of the study suggested that both these procedures improved workers' job performance over baseline levels, but that a combination of the two procedures resulted in the most improvement in job performance.

Summary and Comments on Use of Incentives

As has been seen above, various programs have employed quite a number of incentive procedures to motivate staff members. At the heart of each one was the specification and measurement of staff members' behaviors, residents' behaviors, or both. In some cases the focus of reinforcement was on staff members' behaviors, as such, though in other cases the focus was on resident progress as a criterion for application of incentives to staff members. With simple feedback to staff members being the basic motivating device, most programs also attached some form of social reinforcement to the feedback, such reinforcement coming from official supervisors (including their allies, the research observers), peers, or even the residents themselves. Social reinforcers employed included praise (individually or in groups); letters of recommendation or reprimand; buddy ratings; aide-of-the-week awards; photographs, plaques, and news reports used to publicly recognize individual and group performance; and efforts to foster competition within groups of staff members or between treatment units. Supervisory personnel had the power to give and take more serious back-up reinforcers such as raises, promotions, vacations, assignment to desired shifts, bonus money or the equivalent (given to all or to selected individuals), time off, suspension without pay, and dismissal. Other reinforcers seemed to fall under the heading of "job enrichment." These included progress through hurdles in a staff training program and increased authority to change treatment programs. Finally, in some cases, maintenance of programmatic staff behaviors was supported by the treatment procedures themselves or the recording of them, as when a point recording system was designed to direct staff members' attention to positive rather than negative behaviors of residents.

In all of the experiments or anecdotal accounts summarized above the target behavior was programmatic staff action, and in most of these reports the measure of success was, in fact, a direct measure of staff members' behavior. As logical as the latter procedures may sound, they miss, or largely miss, the main point of staff supervision, which is to effect beneficial change in residents. The underlying assumption of such procedures is that the directors or planners of the treatment program know or suspect they know which procedures will be therapeutic and think that if the treatment staff can be induced to perform these procedures, the residents will change for the better. While not necessarily erroneous, such an assumption can be far wrong in practice. At the least, efforts to provide incentives to staff members should be supplemented by measures of resident response to staff treatment. Few of the reports summarized above provided both kinds of data. A few authors used resident improvement as the criterion for incentives for staff members. Martin, et al. (1973) provided the only study showing a comparison between the two kinds of criteria, and their data supported using resident improvement as the criterion for staff rewards.

One issue here is that at one extreme one could simply give full authority to one's staff members to design and execute treatment programs with individual residents and then reward those staff members whose residents improved. However, if one takes this course, one runs the risk that staff members will not have the relevant information or good supervision necessary to bring about success with residents. One psychologist told the author that if he allowed one of his staff members to choose the form of treatment for residents, then the residents would soon find themselves in the hands of a local astrologer. On the other hand, if one attempts to control all staff members' therapeutic activities, one runs the risk of having a perfectly functioning staff, but poor treatment results.

The solution, it seems to us, is to train one's staff, to offer them periodic retraining or checkouts on procedures, and frequent supervision plus rewards for good performance; but to decentralize responsibility for detailed treatment planning. Staff members could propose treatment plans which could be approved with modifications if indicated by the director, a committee, or by the treatment team as a whole. Then, responsibility for successfully carrying out the approved plan could be given to those staff members who actually carry out the approved treatment program. No staff member would be asked to implement a treatment program that did not meet with his approval. Staff rewards would go to staff members whose residents improved to some preset criterion. With this kind of criterion, staff members might tend to carry out the spirit as well as the letter of the prescribed treatment program. Such procedures might go far toward insuring that staff members both attempt reasonable procedures and do more than just go through the motions of treatment.

CONCLUSIONS

Heller (1972), in his generally pessimistic review of industrial incentive programs, noted that even the best management programs sometimes fail and recommended that ideal management procedures be followed not because of their inevitable success, but simply because they are "right." Our observation is that even the best attempts to train, retrain, and supervise effectively may fail. There is certainly no guarantee that even the most carefully planned treatment program administered by the most competent, well trained, and closely supervised employees will succeed. Failure of a treatment program can undermine the feelings of self-worth and zest of any staff member, no matter how well he performs his job and no matter how much extrinsic reinforcement he gets. Much also depends on the political climate both within the institution and within state and national governments. It is difficult to maintain one's efficiency if one's job is threatened by arbitrary and unreasoned political events.

It is also true that even in the best of situations jobs pale. Bright trainees have been known to reject highly structured treatment programs when given a choice (e.g. Gardner, 1972). The author has heard anecdotal reports that bright, well trained employees in a very successful treatment program for children with behavior problems tended to "burn out" within three to four years. It is possible that the behavioral emphasis on specification of duties, while conducive to effective training and treatment, take some of the mystery from such jobs and eventually bores employees. This is a pessimistic view and probably one that is not warranted in the short run. In fact, behavioral programs tend to be very intricate, not really cut and dried, and replete with challenging failures which tax the ingenuity of staff members. But, even with all this food for thought and action, employees may eventually feel they are just going through old motions. If this feeling is pervasive in a treatment program, there may be something wrong with the program itself that can be changed, but if this feeling is common only to "old" employees, some employment counseling may be in order either to shift them to different duties within the established program, or to move them to other programs or even to a completely different kind of work. This recommendation applies to all staff levels within a program.

This chapter has focused on training and motivating staff members within residential treatment programs. Sophisticated readers will undoubtedly be aware of the main problem associated with any such treatment program, that is, recidivism. The pessimism in our field about getting behaviors trained in residential settings to generalize to the "real world" is justified. The obvious solution is to do our therapy in the real world to begin with. If that is done, then the problem of providing good staff training and supervision takes on a whole new dimension. Paraprofessionals working in the community will have to understand what they are up to and certainly cannot be mere automatons. On-the-job training will have to shift from the comfortable, air-conditioned, institution to vagarious community situations. Supervision will become more difficult, but still could occur on a spot-check basis. It is in this kind of situation that using resident progress as the criterion for awarding staff incentives would come into its own, for constant surveillance would become an impossibility. Periodic assessments of client status would be a possible and possibly quite effective means of remotely supervising paraprofessional community workers.

REFERENCES

Atthowe, J. M., Jr.: Token economies come of age. *Behav Ther,* 4:646, 1973.

Ayllon, T., and Azrin, N.: *The Token Economy: A Motivational System for Therapy and Rehabilitation.* New York, Appleton, 1968.

Barton, E. S.; Guess, D.; Garcia, E., and Baer, D. M.: Improvement of retardates' mealtime behaviors by timeout procedures using multiple baseline techniques. *J Appl Behav Anal, 3*:77, 1970.

Bricker, W. A.; Morgan, D. G., and Grabowski, J. G.: Development and maintenance of a behavior modification repertoire of cottage attendants through TV feedback. *Am J Ment Defic, 77*:128, 1972.

Carlaw, R. W.: The development of interaction as an approach to training. *Public Health Rep, 85*:754, 1970.

Colman, A. D., and Boren, J. J.: An information system for measuring patient behavior and its use by staff. *J Appl Behav Anal, 2*:207, 1969.

Cone, J. D., and Sheldon, S. S.: Training Behavior Modifiers: Getting It Going with Remote Auditory Prompting. Paper presented at the annual American Psychological Convention, Montreal, Canada, August 1973.

Cossairt, A.; Hall, R. V., and Hopkins, B. L.: The effects of experimenter's instructions, feedback, and praise on teacher praise and student attending behavior. *J Appl Behav Anal, 6*:89, 1973.

D'Augelli, A. R.: Strategies for the Comprehensive Evaluation of Training Programs for Nonprofessional Service Workers. Paper presented at the annual meeting of the American Psychological Association, Montreal, Canada, August 1973.

Distefano, M .K., Jr., and Pryer, M. W.: Job analysis of paraprofessional psychiatric nursing personnel. *Journal Supplement Abstract Service Catalog of Selected Documents in Psychology, 3*:92, 1973.

Favell, J. E.: Reduction of Staff Tardiness by a Feedback Procedure. Paper presented at the annual meeting of the American Psychological Association, Montreal, Canada, 1973.

Fein, M.: For workers, a productivity incentive. *New York Times,* February 17, 1974, p. 16.

Friedlander, F., and Brown, L. D.: Organization development. *Ann Rev Psychol, 25*:313, 1974.

Gardner, J. M.: Teaching behavior modification to nonprofessionals. *J Appl Behav Anal, 5*:517, 1972.

Glaser, E. M., and Taylor, S. H.: Factors influencing the success of applied research. *Am Psychol, 28*:140, 1973.

Goldstein, A. P.; Cohen, R.; Blake, G., and Walsh, W.: The effects of modeling and social class structuring in paraprofessional psychotherapist training. *J Nerv Ment Dis, 153*:47, 1971.

Goldstein, A. P., and Goedhart, A.: The use of structured learning for empathy enhancement in paraprofessional psychotherapist training. *J Community Psychol, 1*:168, 1973.

Goldstein, A. P., and Sorcher, M.: Changing managerial behavior by applied learning techniques. *Training and Development Journal,* American Society for Training and Development, Madison, Wisconsin, March 1973.

Heller, R.: *The Great Executive Dream.* New York, Dell, 1972.

Hermann, J. A.; de Montes, A. I.; Dominquez, B.; Montes, F., and Hopkins, B. L.: Effects of bonuses for punctuality on the tardiness of industrial workers. *J Appl Behav Anal, 6*:563, 1973.

Katz, R. C.; Johnson, C. A., and Gelfand, S.: Modifying the dispensing of reinforcers: Some implications for behavior modification with hospitalized patients. *Behav Ther, 3*:579, 1972.

Krasner, L.: Behavoir modification ,token economies, and training in clinical psycholgy. In Neuringer, C., and Michael, J. L. (Eds.): *Behavior Modification in Clinical Psychology.* New York, Appleton, 1970.

Loeber, R.: Engineering the behavioral engineer. *J Appl Behav Anal, 4*:321, 1971.

Martin, G. L.; McDonald, L., and Murrell, M.: Developing and Maintaining Behavior Modification Skills of Psychiatric Nurses, Aides, and Attendants Working with Institutionalized Retardates. Paper presented at the annual convention of the American Psychological Association, Montreal, Canada, August 1973.

Panyan, M.; Boozer, H., and Morris, N.: Feedback to attendants as a reinforcer for applying operant techniques. *J Appl Behav Anal, 3*:1, 1970.

Patterson, R.; Cooke, C. ,and Liberman, R. P.: Reinforcing the reinforcers: A method of supplying feedback to nursing personnel. *Behav Ther, 3*:444, 1972.

Paul, G. L., and McInnis, T. L.: Attitudinal changes associated with two approaches to training mental health technicians in milieu and social-learning programs. *J Consult Clin Psychol, 42*:21, 1974.

Paul, G. L.; McInnis, T. L., and Mariotto, M. J.: Objective performance outcomes associated with two approaches to training mental health technicians in milieu and social-learning programs. *J Abnormal Psychol, 82*:523, 1973.

Phillips, E. L.; Phillips, E. A.; Wolf, M. M., and Fixsen, D. L.: Achievement Place: Development of the elected manager system. *J Appl Behav Anal, 6*:541, 1973.

Pomerleau, O. F.; Bobrove, P. H., and Smith, R. H.: Rewarding psychiatric aides for the behavioral improvement of assigned patients. *J Appl Behav Anal, 6*:383, 1973.

Pommer, D. A., and Streedbeck, D.: Motivating staff performance in an operant learning program for children. *J Appl Behav Anal, 7*:217, 1974.

Rappaport, J.; Gross, T., and Lepper, C.: Modeling, sensitivity training and instruction: Implications for the training of college student volunteers and for outcome research. *J Consult Clin Psychol, 40*:99, 1973.

Smith, R. C., and Carlin, J.: Behavior modification using interlocking reinforcement on a short-term psychiatric ward. *Arch Gen Psychiatry*, 27:386, 1972.

Watson, L. S.; Gardner, J. M., and Sanders, C.: Shaping and maintaining behavior modification skills in staff members in an MR institution: Columbus State Institute Behavior Modification Program. *Ment Retard*, 9:39, 1971.

Wolf, M. M.; Giles, D. K., and Hall, R. V.: Experiments with token reinforcement in a remedial classroom. *Behav Res Ther*, 6:51, 1968.

Chapter IV

SHAPING AND MAINTAINING BEHAVIOR MODIFICATION SKILLS IN STAFF USING CONTINGENT REINFORCEMENT TECHNIQUES

LUKE S. WATSON, JR., PH.D.

T HIS CHAPTER IS concerned with *practical* applications of contingent reinforcement techniques to shaping and maintaining behavior modification skills in staff in behavior modification programs. Practical contingencies include various types of recognition from supervisors, special privileges, time off from work, and money (whenever it is feasible to use cash in a given bureaucratic system). The population to which the term "staff" refers consists of direct-care staff in residential institutions, teachers, teacher aides, and parents. The contents of the chapter will be a discussion of the *requirements* for setting up a contingent reinforcement system for staff, a summary of a complete staff reinforcement system, and some rather limited (and not rigorous) supporting data to justify the major points.

One of the greatest deficiencies in most behavior modification programs is the lack of a well-developed staff reinforcement system. Because of this problem, these programs usually are severely compromised. Staff in schools, institutions, or mental health centers fail to train clients, i.e. students, residents, or patients regularly, and frequently do not carry out training procedures correctly. As a result client improvement or progress is minimal. This problem is particularly grave in residential institutions for the mentally retarded or mentally ill. When viewed in

69

conjunction with the absence of the necessary supportive administrative, and data systems (that will be proposed shortly), the lack of adequate staff reinforcement systems probably is responsible for a majority of the client training problems that occur in behavior modification programs.

In order to provide an effective staff reinforcement system, three requirements must be satisfied: An *administrative system* that permits staff contingent reinforcement must be created, a *data system* that adequately tracks staff performance must be instituted, and an *in-service training program* that teaches staff the requisite behavior modification skills must be developed. Once these systems exist, it is then possible to effectively reinforce staff. These three systems will be considered before progressing to the problem of staff reinforcement. Finally and most importantly, none of these systems can be developed independently of the others. *Each must be an integral part of a total, synchronized behavior modification program.* Each system should be developed or deduced from a broad set of behavioral objectives which constitute the major purpose, goal, or thrust of the program. This is the point at which any behavior modification program should begin.

OVERALL PROGRAM GOALS

During the period 1968-1973, two behavior modification programs were developed at Columbus State Institute.* One was designed to teach compliance, self-help, language, motor coordination, and academic and social recreational skills to severely and profoundly retarded* residents in the institution. The other was designed to teach parents of psychotic and retarded children

---

* The two programs were supported by a Hospital Improvement Project Grant (#51-P-700-80), a Hospital In-service Training Grant (#52-P-70174), a Mental Retardation Facilities Staffing Grant (#1-H01-MR-08181), and a DDA Grant from the State of Ohio (#1971-6).

* Severely and profoundly mentally retarded fall in the class of retardates with IQ's of thirty-five or less. Heber, R. F.: *A Manual on Terminology in Mental Retardation,* second edition. *Monograph Supplement* to the *American Journal of Mental Deficiency* (Willimantic, Connecticut, American Association on Mental Deficiency, 1961).

in the community how to develop compliance in their children and teach them self-help, language, social-recreational skills, motor coordination, and academic skills—and prevent them from ever being admitted to an institution such as Columbus State Institute. The first step taken in designing these programs was to identify a *broad set of behavioral goals or objectives.* The major goal of the program for residents at Columbus State Institute was to provide them with the necessary skills to allow them to return to the community and adapt satisfactorily to this type of life. Since they were severely retarded, the target community life style was to have them live in a semi-independent community living situation and be employed by a sheltered workshop. The major goal for psychotic and retarded children in the community program utilizing parents as trainers was to enable them to adapt to life at home with their parents and siblings, be admitted to a community special educational academic program, and be accepted by the principal, teachers, and students.

Once these broad goals were identified for the two programs, the next step was to identify all of the behaviors the resident or child would need to achieve the broad major program goals. The goals were listed in six categories: elimination of undesirable behavior and compliance, motor coordination, and self-help; language, academic, and social-recreational skills. All behaviors were identified for each category, and criteria for determining when each behavior was satisfactorily acquired were eventually developed. An illustration of the total set of goals identified for the community behavior modification program can be found in Table IV-I.

The total list of specific behavioral goals needed to meet the broad program objectives summarized in Table IV-I was called the "Model Child." This list of goals presumably identified all behaviors a retarded or psychotic child would need to be-behaviorally approximate a relatively normal child of a similar chronological age. Although such an individual would not have the same "cognitive" skills as a normal child of his age, once he acquired all of the skills summarized in the Model Child, he would appear to be similar to the normal child to the casual observer and should be able to make a satisfactory adjustment to

TABLE IV-I

MODEL CHILD SCHEMATIC SUMMARY OF TRAINING GOALS
OR TARGET BEHAVIORS SELECTED FOR CHILDREN IN
CHILDREN'S BEHAVIOR MODIFICATION PROGRAM

SELF-HELP SKILLS	
Skill	*Target Behaviors*
Eating	Can sit at table and eat neatly with spoon or fork (or equivalent to age level).
	Lack of Inappropriate Behavior: Does not jump up from table until meal is completed; does not throw food or eat with his fingers; does not take food from someone else's plate, scream or cry; does not chew food with mouth open; does not swallow solid food without chewing it; does not pound eating utensils on the table; does not spin plate, drop it or throw it.
Drinking	Can drink neatly from an appropriate size cup or glass held in one hand (unless younger than age three). *Lack of Inappropriate Behavior*: Does not pound cup on table, drop it or throw cup or its contents; does not place fingers or hands in cup or blow bubbles; does not put food, napkins, utensils, clothing or other objects in cup; does not spin cup; does not spit contents or gargle.
Undressing	Can remove pants, shirt, coat, dress, underpants, undershirt or other undergarments (with or without buttons, zippers or snaps), socks and shoes (either with buckles or laces) without assistance or supervision (or equivalent to his age level).
	Lack of Inappropriate Behavior: Does not damage garments when removing them; does not throw them on the floor and leave them.
Dressing	Can put on pants, shirt, coat, dress or underclothing (with or without buttons, zippers, or snaps), socks and shoes (either with buckles or laces) appropriately without assistance or supervision (or equivalent to his age level).
	Lack of Inappropriate Behavior: Does not damage garments when putting them on.
Toileting	Will locomote to toilet when elimination is impending without being cued; removes lower clothing appropriately; sits appropriately (unless male who is urinating); urinates or defecates into toilet bowl; wipes appropriately when elimination is completed without using an excessive amount of paper, deposits paper in toilet, flushes, pulls up underpants and/or pants, and washes hands and dries them (or equivalent to his age level).
	Lack of Inappropriate Behavior: Does not play in toilet bowl, nor smear feces nor drink from bowl, nor urinate on tank or floor or bathtub; does not stop up toilet with excessive toilet paper or other objects.

TABLE IV-I (Continued)

SELF-HELP SKILLS (Continued)	
Skill	*Target Behaviors*
Bathing	Can fill tub or turn on shower and adjust water temperature; can soap washcloth and bathe all parts of body, rinses and dries; and can allow water to drain from tub (or equivalent to his age level).
	Lack of Inappropriate Behavior: Does not drink bath water, stop up drain with foreign objects; and does not flood the bathroom.
Toothbrushing	Applies appropriate amount of toothpaste to toothbrush, brushes all surfaces appropriately, rinses out mouth and rinses off toothbrush, and returns toothbrush to receptable (or equivalent to age level).
	Lack of Inappropriate Behavior: Does not squeeze excessive toothpaste onto toothbrush, bite toothpaste tube or damage tube; does smear toothpaste on sink, mirror or other inappropriate areas; does not splatter with toothbrush; does not swallow toothpaste; does not gag himself; and does not throw toothbrush.
Gross Locomotor Development	Can walk down steps one foot per tread, skips, jumps and runs without inappropriate posture or mannerisms (or equivalent to age level).
Fine Motor Development	Can manipulate small objects with hands and fingers using thumbs; can place puzzle pieces in formboards, pegs in pegboards, lace shoes, snap, buckle and tie shoes, and color with crayons and cut with scissors; can throw and catch a ball with two hands (or equivalent to age level).

ABSENCE OF UNDESIRABLE BEHAVIOR	
Elimination of Temper Tantrums	Does not cry, scream, run about, lie on the floor and kick, flail his arms, etc.
Elimination of Destructive Behavior	Does not damage toys, furniture or other inanimate objects.
Elimination of Self-Abusive Behavior	Does not beat or slap his head with his hands; beat his head against floor, wall or furniture; bite himself; pull out his hair, etc.
Elimination of Abusiveness to Others	Does not hit, bite or scratch parents, siblings, peers, or staff, neither does he strike them with inanimate objects, spit on them, nor pull their hair.
Elimination of Stereotyped or Ritualistic Behavior	Does not rock, sway, or gesture symbolically in a repetitive manner; does not move his fingers in front of his face repetitively; does not twirl or spin objects; does not engage in any other bizarre, repetitive behavior.

TABLE IV-I (Continued)

ABSENCE OF UNDESIRABLE BEHAVIOR (Continued)	
Skill	*Target Behaviors*
Elimination of Smearing Feces	Does not smear feces on himself, others, walls, floors or furniture.
Elimination of Lack of Eye Contact	Looks at people when they look at him or talk to him or ask him to look at them.
Elimination of Failure to Look at Task	Looks at task he is engaging in; such as completing a puzzle or throwing and catching a ball.
Elimination of Short Attention Span	Can work at a task without interruptions up to 40 minutes.
Elimination of Hyperactivity	Does not constantly run or pace about the house or school.
Elimination of Constantly Getting into Things	Does not strew contents of pantry, kitchen drawers, bathroom cabinets, etc.
Elimination of Uncooperativeness	Does what he is told to do promptly.
Elimination of Lack of Motivation	Active, interested in a variety of tasks and activities, responsive to a variety of edible, manipulatable and social reinforcements.
Elimination of Eating Objects That Are Not Food Items	Does not eat string, feces, sticks, rocks, toys, etc.
Elimination of Ignoring Other Children	Looks at children when they are within view, approaches them, talks to them, and smiles at them, and displays affection for them; shows affection for siblings and friends.
Elimination of Ignoring Parents	Looks at parents when they are within view, approaches them, talks to them, and smiles at them, and displays affection for them.
Elimination of Ignoring Other Adults	Looks at adults when they are within view, approaches them, talks to them, and smiles at them.
Elimination of Resistance to Change of Routine	Does not cry, scream or otherwise object when furniture, food on plate or other items are rearranged.
Elimination of Resistance to Being Interrupted at a Task	Does not cry, scream, have a tantrum, or otherwise object when asked to stop a task or activity he is engaging in.
Elimination of Resistance to Being Held or Cuddled	Does not cry, scream, stiffen or push away when parents, relatives, friends or siblings attempt to hold or cuddle him.

TABLE IV-I (Continued)

ABSENCE OF UNDESIRABLE BEHAVIOR (Continued)

Skill	Target Behaviors
Elimination of Taking Off Clothes Inappropriately	Does not remove clothing in public places or in home other than in bedroom or bathroom or at toileting time, bathtime or bedtime.
Elimination of Running Away	Does not run away from home or school or from parents in public places.
Elimination of Profane or Hostile Language	Does not express profane or hostile language toward others inappropriately.
Elimination of Misbehaving in Public	Does not refuse to obey in stores or exhibit temper tantrums or behave in other inappropriate ways.

LANGUAGE SKILLS

Imitates	Models trainer or other children upon command the first time when a novel behavior is introduced (or equivalent to age level).
Responsiveness to Sound	Shows orientation response to a sound that occurs out of line of vision and can discriminate sounds (or equivalent to age level).
Receptive Language: Single Words	Responds appropriately to or indicates understanding of approximately 2,500 words (or equivalent to age level).
Receptive Language: Commands	Responds appropriately to approximately 250 commands (or equivalent to age level).
Concepts	Understands prepositional concepts; concepts of time, distance, shape, quantity, location, texture, weight, color; and societal value judgments (or equivalent to age level).
Expressive Language: Single Words	Can say approximately 1,200 words (or equivalent to age level).
Expressive Language: Sentence Complexity Used to Make Demands or Requests	Uses sentences utilizing 6-10 words on the average (or equivalent to age level).
Expressive Language: Sentence Complexity Used to Relate Experiences	Uses sentences utilizing 8-10 words on the average (or equivalent to age level).
Quality of Articulation	Omits, distorts or substitutes "r" sounds, "s" sounds and "z" sounds (or equivalent to age level).
Words Used Appropriately	Uses speech appropriate to situation (or equivalent to age level).

TABLE IV-I (Continued)

EDUCATIONAL SKILLS

Skill	Target Behaviors
Seat Work	Can sit at a table with peers and carry out a structured task without interruptions up to 20 minutes and without disturbing neighbors—with limited supervision.
Seat Work	Can sit at a table with peers and carry out a semistructured task without interruption up to 20 minutes and without disturbing neighbors—with limited supervision.
Group Tasks	Can interact appropriately with a group of 8-10 in a common task.
Knows His Way Around	Does not get lost going to and from school or from classroom to bathroom, lunchroom, or playground.

SOCIAL-RECREATIONAL SKILLS

Solitary Play	Engages in a variety of structured activities appropriately, e.g. works formboard puzzles, plays a solitary lotto game, completes pegboard designs, or swings in a swing, up to 30 minutes (or equivalent to age level) with limited supervision.
Solitary Play	Engages in a variety of semistructured activities appropriately, e.g. rocks on a rocking horse, plays with a toy truck, colors in a coloring book or roller-skates up to 45 minutes with liimted supervision (or equivalent to age level).
Solitary Play	Engages in a variety of unstructured activities, e.g. plays with a doll, draws a picture or plays in a sandbox appropriately up to 15 minutes with limited supervision (or equivalent to age level).
Cooperative Play	Engages in a variety of structured activities appropriately, e.g. works puzzles, plays a lotto game or dominoes, swings or bowls with up to four other children for 25 minutes (or equivalent to age level).
Cooperative Play	Engages in a variety of semistructured activities appropriately, e.g. plays on teeter-totters, throws and catches a ball, and plays Simon Says with up to four other children for 35 minutes (or equivalent to age level).
Cooperative Play	Engages in a variety of unstructured activities appropriately, e.g. plays in a sandbox, plays with a doll, plays house or cowboys and Indians with up to four other children for 20 minutes (or equivalent to age level).
Conversation	Engages in dialogue with up to three other children for up to 20 minutes (or equivalent to age level).
Spontaneous Horse Play	Engages in spontaneous horse play for approximately 10 minutes (or equivalent to age level).

TABLE IV-I (Continued)

SOCIAL-RECREATIONAL SKILL (Continued)	
Skill	*Target Behaviors*
Competition	Strives to win at competitive games and appears to enjoy winning; reacts appropriately to losing.
Response to Other Players in Games	Pays attention when another child is taking his turn in a game and smiles, laughs or makes an appropriate vocal response when another player scores.
Initiative	Initiates conversation and games with other children.

the community life-style identified in the major program goal. After the total list of behaviors needed to satisfy the overall program goal was completed, it then was possible to proceed with the development of the *administrative system, data system, in-service training system,* and *staff reinforcement system.* These four systems were deduced from or followed from the Model Child or list of total specific behaviors. The major point is that without first identifying the overall program goals and then determining all specific behaviors clients would need to satisfy the broad program goals, it was not possible to functionally generate the other systems necessary to develop an integrated/synchronized set of systems that would be needed to set up an effective behavior modification program.

ADMINISTRATIVE SYSTEM

The administrative system needed to permit an effective staff reinforcement system should be designed with one criterion in mind. It must be possible to determine when a staff member is training clients correctly (and also to identify specific inadequacies in staff performance). If this criterion is not met, it is not possible to use contingent reinforcement procedures effectively with staff. Since behavior modification programs with the mentally retarded and mentally ill are primarily concerned with acquisition of skills by clients, the two most relevant categories of staff behaviors are patient or client training and data collection. We found from the outset that a particular type of administrative model was needed to allow daily patient or resident training and record keeping in residential institutions, particularly a large institution (with a resident population exceeding 500).

Administrative Model

This model should be based on a training or *rehabilitation* orientation as opposed to a *custodial* treatment orientation. An Educational Unit System with an administrative model of the type summarized in Figure IV-1 is an ideal model. The unit system permits (behaviorally) homogeneous groupings of residents which facilitate training. There are three key administrative positions that control client treatment in this particular model. These are the superintendent, the program director, and the director of research and training. The success or failure of any training program is primarily dependent upon them. In this model, these three positions are occupied by persons with a habilitative orientation and/or education. They usually hold degrees in special education or psychology. The important factor that requires these three types of positions is that they will maintain *training* as a first priority and *custodial treatment* as a second priority, something that is necessary if effective habilitative programs are to function. Second- or third-priority training programs rarely succeed in institutional settings because of a chronic shortage of staff and other resources.

The other key positions in this administrative model are the coordination/evaluation positions. Notice there is one overall coordinator/evaluator who is directly responsible to the superintendent. Then the program director has one directly responsible to him as does each unit director. There also is such a position in the research and training department directly responsible to the director of research and training. The key functions performed by these positions is to maintain synchronization among all habilitative programs to produce a total integrated/coordinated effort within the institution's habilitative system. To do this, these persons have a feedback system based on an evaluative procedure (that will be considered later). The function performed by the coordinator/evaluator at the unit level is to obtain

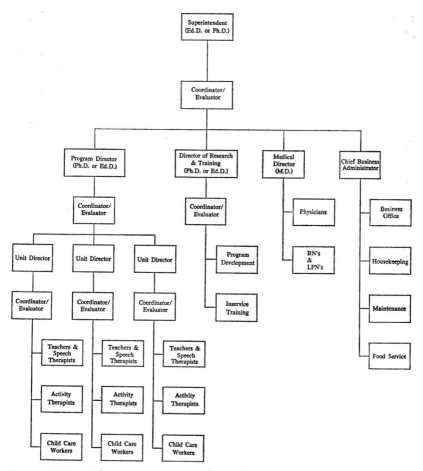

Figure IV-1. Schematic summary of an Educational Unit System administrative model.

feedback from and coordinate all training activities of all teachers, speech therapists, activity therapists, and child-care aides. If the various staff members are not carrying out their training functions effectively, he determines why, i.e. troubleshoots, and gets them back on the track. The coordinator/evaluator at the program-director level obtains feedback from the three unit-level co-ordinator/evaluators and sees that all unit training staff are working toward the overall goal agreed upon for the institution in a synchronized manner. He also performs interrater reliability checks on the three unit-level coordinator/evaluators.

The coordinator/evaluator in the research and training department department obtains feedback on the effectiveness of the in-service training program and any new client training programs that are developed. He is particularly interested in determining whether the in-service training program and client training programs effectively carry over to the living units or cottages and the schools and recreational areas—i.e. whether the programs generalize to the areas where they are designed to function. If they do not, his job is to troubleshoot the problem and correct it. He also provides a reliability or credibility check on the unit-level coordinator/evaluators. The last coordinator/evaluator is responsible to the superintendent. His job is to obtain feedback from the coordinator/evaluator directly responsible to the program director and the director of research and training. He coordinates the efforts of the two departments and keeps them working in synchrony. He too performs reliability and credibility checks on these two coordinator/evaluators. All of these coordinator/evaluators ensure that all programs work effectively and efficiently. Without them, it is virtually impossible to operate a comprehensive, intensive, multidisciplinary behavior modification program successfully.

The coordinator/evaluators can either have administrative line authority over everyone beneath them or simply provide feedback to their superiors, depending upon which of the two alternatives is most compatible with the administrative system in the particular organization. If the superintendent, program director, and unit directors are very busy, it may be useful to give administrative line authority to the coordinator/evaluators and simply allow them to control all training activities. However, if the different administrators prefer to run their own departments and make all administrative decisions, then the coordinator/evaluators can be limited to providing feedback to the administrators.

In essence, the evaluator/coordinator's role is twofold: to detect client training problems by means of the feedback he receives from the data supplied by other staff and to see that the problems are corrected as soon as possible. Both functions are essential. Without a satisfactory detection system (data system), he would not be able to identify the training problems. Without corrective action, detection of problems is a useless exercise, and the training programs may be compromised.

It is very difficult to carry out regular client training in certain kinds of administrative models, particularly the custodial administrative model of the type usually found in the medical model residential institution (see Fig. IV-2). Such a model is designed primarily to provide custodial treatment to patients. The two key administrative staff members, the superintendent and the director of nursing, are trained primarily to provide medical, psychiatric, and/or nursing treatment to patients. They typically subscribe to the "disease" orientation toward mental

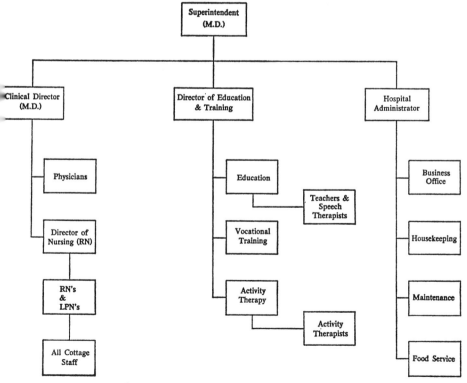

Figure IV-2.   Schematic summary of a custodial administrative model.

retardation and mental illness, and are not trained in psycho-educational procedures that are relevant to carrying out training programs with their residents or patients. Training usually is a low-priority item in this administrative system and usually is carried out only after all custodial obligations are satisfied. Their general orientation is basically incompatible with the behavior modification approach. (For a detailed discussion of this problem, see Ullman and Krasner, 1965; and Kugel and Wolfensberger, 1969.)

Accountability/Responsibility

One key factor relevant to staff reinforcement in an administrative system is an effective accountability/responsibility system. Each staff member's responsibilities should be clearly delineated. It also should be clear to which supervisors each staff member is accountable. Again, this is a particularly important consideration in a residential institution.

Using our behavior modification program for residents at Columbus State Institute as an example, clearcut delineations of responsibility and accountability were set up for direct-care staff. They are summarized in Figure IV-3 and Table IV-II. As

TABLE IV-II
SPECIFIC RESPONSIBILITIES OF BEHAVIOR
MODIFICATION TECHNICIANS

Training	tion and overall	*Housekeeping*	*Medical*
1. Get children up	training and care	1. Supervise work-	1. Resident
2. Toileting and	of residents	ing girls. If	treatments
toilet training	*Administration*	they are not	2. Chart medical
3. Washing and	1. Communicate	present, assume	records
grooming	with all staff	their duties.	
4. Dressing train-	about training	2. Special	
ing or requiring	of residents	laundry	
residents to dress	to insure	3. Order and	
5. Bib for all meals	consistency of	mend clothing,	
6. Supervise free	training	order pressing	
play	2. Order supplies		
7. Eating training	3. Maintain ward		
for all meals	in absence of		
8. Education	charge and		
programs	supervisors		
9. Special training			
for individual			
residents, e.g.			
head-banging			
10. Data collection			
11. Bath training			
12. General observa-			

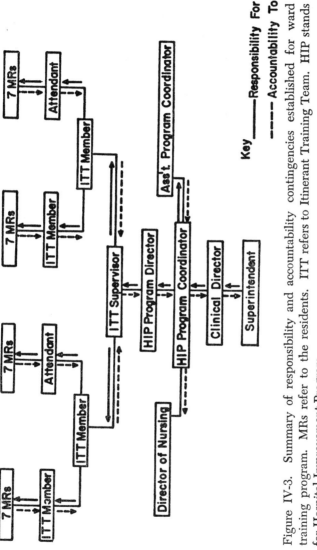

Figure IV-3.   Summary of responsibility and accountability contingencies established for ward training program. MRs refer to the residents.   ITT refers to Itinerant Training Team.   HIP stands for Hospital Improvement Program.

Figure IV-3 indicates, each direct-care staff member was responsible to *only* one supervisor. The main purpose was to limit the "two-three-or-more-bosses" system that invariably creates confusion within the chain of command and prevents a determination of *who told whom to do what*. It is virtually impossible for a staff member to follow the dictates of two or more supervisors. He must ultimately play one off against the other to protect himself.

With regard to responsibility, each direct care-staff member was responsible for certain residents (as indicated in Fig. IV-3). If the resident showed progress, the supervisor knew who to credit for it. On the other hand, if a resident was walking around soiled or wet or unattended, it also was clear to the supervisor which staff member was negligent in her duties.

Table IV-II summarizes the other total spectrum of responsibilities of direct-care staff in the Columbus State Institute Program. They had administrative, housekeeping and medical, as well as training duties. Each staff member knew all of her responsibilities, and it also was clear who took over for her on her days off. An interesting note is that staff participated in deciding just what their duties should be in order to take care of both custodial and training requirements; i.e. on the ward, management by staff participation was employed. This presumably increased their cooperativeness and support of the program.

The main responsibilities of supervisors were to give subordinate staff recognition or reinforcement for training residents and to troubleshoot problems in daily resident training and custodial work assignments. They were not supposed to play the traditional, authoritorian-custodial-institutional supervisor role. The specific reinforcement contingencies employed by supervisors will be considered later.

A realistic daily resident training schedule (see Table IV-III) was also another administrative procedure that appeared to contribute to an effective administrative system. This schedule was set up by the entire program staff, i.e. the program administrators, supervisors, and trainers working in collaboration. It was found that, without such a schedule, training and other

TABLE IV-III

DAILY WARD SCHEDULE FOR RESIDENTS

COLUMBUS STATE INSTITUTE BEHAVIOR MODIFICATION PROGRAM

6:00- 7:30	Residents up, toileted, dressing skills carried out
7:30- 8:30	Free play, prepared for breakfast (must be dressed to have bib)
8:30- 9:00	Breakfast
9:00- 9:30	Toileting and free play
9:30-10:30	Ward programs (educational and recreational)
10:30-11:30	Free play, prepared for lunch (must be involved in activity to have bib)
11:30-12:00	Lunch (must say grace)
12:00-12:30	Toileting
12:30- 2:30	Extra training (as needed)
	Outside activities, walks, play equipment, etc.
	Free play
2:30- 3:30	Ward programs (educational and recreational)
3:30- 4:00	Toileting
4:00- 5:00	Free play
5:00- 5:30	Dinner (must say grace)
5:30- 6:00	Toileting
6:00- 8:00	Outside (if weather permits), free play, extra training as needed
8:00- 9:00	Dressing skills, grooming, toothbrushing
9:00- 9:30	Bathing training and to bed

functions (see Table IV-II) were never carried out on any regular basis.

DATA SYSTEM

Program coordinators, administrators, and supervisors cannot function effectively without feedback. This is accomplished through a simple, effective-reliable data system. Such a system should not only be easy to use to obtain the *relevant* data and be reliable, but it also should be extremely economical, both in terms of the time it takes for the trainer to record the client's performance and also with regard to the time it takes supervisors, coordinators, and administrators to interpret the data summaries they receive.

Two sets of evaluative instruments were developed: one to survey broad categories of behavior, e.g. self-help skills, and the other to assess specific training programs, e.g. toilet training or dressing pants. Program coordinators were primarily concerned

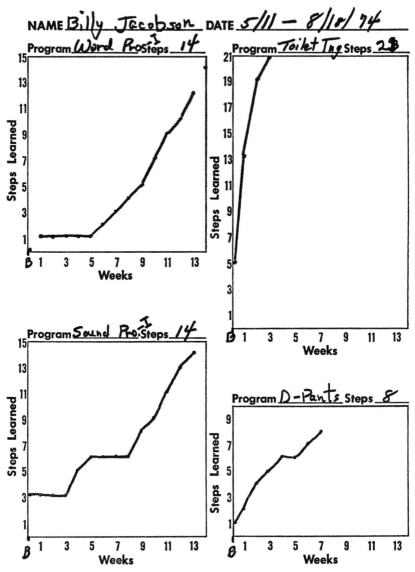

Figure IV-4.   An example of a graph summary sheet.

with using survey instruments to screen residents prior to initiating training (a sample of this type of assessment device can be found in Watson, 1972a on p. 191). Resident training staff or parents usually used specific training program assessment instruments to evaluate progress of residents or children in programs (see Chap. 10 in Watson, 1973).

One of the greatest problems encountered when a large number of clients (30 or more) are enrolled in a program is to review and interpret meaningfully the accumulated data frequently enough to revise specific programs which do not appear sufficiently effective with the client. This problem was handled by developing a graph summary sheet. As Figure IV-4 indicates, all programs summarized with this graph were broken down into steps. Then the relevant data recorded was the number of steps in each training program the client learned each week. So, once a week the graph summary was filled out. Notice the graph can be used for thirteen weeks (or three months). The first entry is the client's pretraining baseline, and each entry in each graph thereafter summarized the client's weekly performance in a training program. This technique provided a succinct summary of the client's performance.

A second feature of this graph summary system relates to quickly identifying (and later troubleshooting) training programs that are not working effectively with particular clients. The slope of the graph easily permits identification of programs that are not producing progress. As long as the slope of the graph moves upward (away from the horizontal), the client is making progress. However, anytime it takes on a horizontal dimension, it becomes immediately obvious progress is not being made in that program. So, if someone is reviewing 25 to 100 program summaries during a given day, all they have to do is quickly scan each data summary and search for horizontal components to the graphs. Once these are identified, relevant staff members can be brought together to determine how to modify the problem program for a particular client. Persons trained in an operant laboratory should find this type of graph particularly appealing.

These graph summaries can be further reduced using a report card (see Fig. IV-5). Periodically (monthly or quarterly) the data from the graph summaries can be reduced even further and recorded on each client's own report card. For progress report purposes, there is a facility or program report card that permits

BMT●
INDIVIDUAL BEHAVIOR MODIFICATION TRAINING SUMMARY

NAME Billy Jacobson
ADDRESS Cottage A
DATE 5-11-74 - 8-18-74

SCORING INSTRUCTIONS:

In each category, place an X for the score the individual acquired on the evaluation instrument. If he learned *less* than half the steps in the program (the number of steps between his baseline and the final step in the program) give an O score; if he learned at least half the steps give him a score of 1; if he learned all the steps, score 2.

Summary Score																		
Date	5/11/74			8/18/74														
Score	0	1	2	0	1	2	0	1	2	0	1	2	0	1	2	0	1	2
Task																		
Toilet Training	X				X													
Utensil Feeding	X				X													
UD - Pants	X				X													
UD - Shirt	X				X													
UD - Socks	X				X													
UD - Shoes	X				X													
Temper Tantrums	X				X													
Sound Production-I	X				X													
Word Production-I	X				X													
Social-Recreation-I	X			X														

© BEHAVIOR MODIFICATION TECHNOLOGY INC., 1974   LITHO IN U.S.A.

Figure IV-5.   An example of an individual report card.

summarizing results of an entire behavior modification program involving a large number of clients on a single piece of paper (see Fig. IV-6).

IN-SERVICE TRAINING

The final system required to permit the use of an effective staff reinforcement system is an in-service training program that

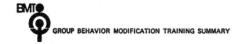

BM **GROUP BEHAVIOR MODIFICATION TRAINING SUMMARY**

FACILITY Wolf Center
ADDRESS Berwyn, Ill.
TOTAL CENSUS 97
DATE 5/11/74 - 8/18/74

SCORING INSTRUCTIONS:
In each category place the number of individuals who have received each score on the Instrument, Individual Behavior Modification Training Summary.

Summary Score Date	5/11/74			8/18/74														
Score / Task	0	1	2	0	1	2	0	1	2	0	1	2	0	1	2	0	1	2
Toilet Training	74	23				97												
Utensil Feeding	62	35				97												
UD - Pants	86	11				97												
UD - Shirt	47	50				97												
UD - Socks	72	13	12			97												
UD - Shoes	73	12	12			97												
Temper Tantrum	11	0	86			97												
Sound Production-I	78	19		4	13	80												
Word Production-I	88	9		7	17	73												
Social-Recreation-I	93	4		2	17	78												

Figure IV-6. An example of a facility report card.

teaches staff the relevant behavior modification skills. Again, the actual characteristics of such a program are deduced or determined from the broad program objectives and the list of specific program goals, e.g. the Model Child. An effective behavior modification in-service training program should teach three sets of skills: (1) how to supervise subordinates using a contingent reinforcement approach, (2) how to use the data systems employed in the program, and (3) how to train residents, patients, or clients.

The system we developed has been used effectively with (or has been standardized with) over 800 psychologists, speech therapists, teachers, parents, nurses, and residential institution direct-care staff. It consists of an academic phase and a practicum followed by a four-month internship period. The academic phase of training is designed to teach staff how to conceptualize the behavior (or "psychodynamics") of their charges in behavior modification terms. It is also during academic training that they receive their initial experiences with data collection. Academic training is broken down into ten units. Each unit consists of a reading assignment in a textbook written specifically for these kinds of students (Watson, 1973), followed by a true-false/fill-in-the-blank examination to assess the student's understanding of the reading assignment. The student must make a 90-percent raw score to meet criterion on this exam. Class begins each day with the examination. Then students are introduced to the second part of the unit: a 35-mm slide accompanied lecture. The lecture illustrates and supplements the material covered in the reading assignment. At the end of the lecture, the student is given an essay examination to assess her understanding of the lecture. Again, the criterion for passing the exam is 90 percent. The essay exam is followed by a discussion of the day's course content. All students participate in the lecture. Students go through one two-hour academic unit a day for a total of ten days. Thus, academic training requires twenty hours to complete.

The practicum involves a book of structured training programs (Watson, 1972a), three movies on self-help, language and social-recreational skill training (Watson, 1972b, c and d), and role playing or initially tutored training sequences. The student is initially assigned the chapter on teaching self-help skills in the book of training programs. After reading the chapter she sees the movie on self-help skill training, and after the movie, she is asked to model what she saw, either with another student in a role-playing sequence or with her own child if she is a parent trainee. While she models, she is assessed by staff using a Training Proficiency Scale, a forty-four-item rating scale designed to shape behavior modification training proficiency (Gardner, et al., 1970; and Watson, 1972a and 1974). The student must meet a 95-percent correct criterion before moving on to the next two practicums: language and social recreation. These last two units are taught using the same procedure described for the first practicum. It takes approximately ten hours to complete practicum training. At the completion of practicum training, the student begins a four-month internship. For a more detailed discussion of this program, see Watson, et al. (1971), and Watson and Bassinger (in press).

Supporting data that demonstrates the effectiveness of the in-service training program are summarized in Figure IV-7, the results of an in-service training program evaluation conducted with a group of parents. This study was designed to assess the relative effectiveness of the academic phase of the program and the practicum. Three parents were used as subjects. Three topics in academic training were assessed: reinforcement, shaping, and stimulus control. Three phases of practicum training also were evaluated: self-help skill training, language training, and social-recreational skill training. In addition, the effects of showing movies were compared with actual, tutored, feedback training in using the Training Proficiency Scale. True-false/fill-in-the-bank test scores were used to assess academic performance, and scores from the Training Proficiency Scale were used to evaluate practicum performance. The main findings were that academic training influenced academic performance but had little influence on performance in practicum. Practicum training was the primary factor influencing performance in practicum, and seeing a movie of someone else training was not as effective for developing criterion-level performance as tutored feedback from the Training Proficiency Scale.

STAFF REINFORCEMENT

Once the administrative, data, and in-service training systems are developed, it is possible to implement a staff reinforcement system. The administrative and data systems make it possible to determine whether staff have met specific reinforcement con-

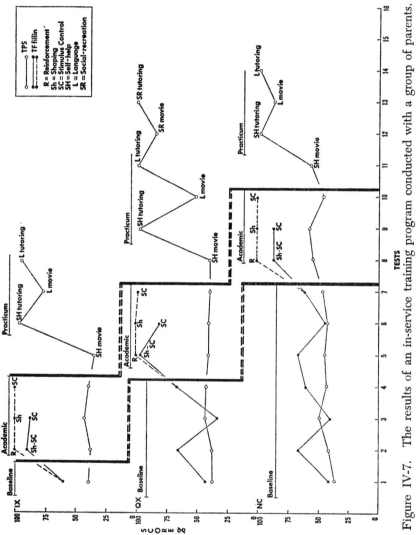

Figure IV-7. The results of an in-service training program conducted with a group of parents.

tingencies, and the in-service training program teaches staff the crucial contingencies that should be met in a client training program. The specific staff reinforcement contingencies should be deduced from the detailed program goals, e.g. the Model Child. The four contingencies we have used for delivering reinforcement to staff in our institutional and community programs were the following:

1. staff are observed training clients correctly;
2. staff are observed recording data on client performance correctly;
3. the data show the client has made progress in the program; and
4. direct observation of the client shows he has made progress in the program.

There were three general types of reinforcement used with staff in the two behavior modification programs:

1. recognition or attention;
2. time off; and
3. money.

Certainly, recognition or attention can be used regardless of the constraints imposed by a municipal, state, or federal bureaucracy. All supervisory staff in our two behavior modification programs used recognition or attention to reinforce staff for satisfying any of the four reinforcement contingencies.* This was accomplished by supervisors observing staff and reinforcing them whenever one of the four contingencies was met. Supervisory staff at Columbus State Institute were working clinicians, and usually trained residents along with subordinate staff. They supervised staff (and reinforced them) as they trained residents. Whenever a home training specialist made a home visit in our community program, she always checked the parent's data for the previous week of training and directly observed her training.

In addition to on-the-spot recognition, staff were given two other kinds of verbal reinforcement. During weekly staff meetings, they were given recognition for having made a significant behavioral change in a particular resident. The resident's name

---

* In order for recognition from supervisors to be an effective staff reinforcement, the supervisors themselves must be competent behavior modifiers.

was announced, and the chairman of the meeting described the nature of the improvement and identified the names of the persons who were training that resident. Pictures of these staff members were then posted on the Recognition Bulletin Board. Also, once a month, an engraved plaque was awarded to the group of staff whose residents had shown the greatest progress during the past thirty days.

Money was used to reinforce institutional staff for maintaining self-help skills in residents once they were acquired. Staff were paid a bonus, on a shift basis, for requiring residents to dress themselves in the morning, eat with utensils and not steal food at mealtime, and shower and put on pajamas prior to going to bed at night.

Time off from work was given primarily for attendance and punctuality. Institutional staff were given half a day off each time they had come to work without being late for twenty-five successive days. This procedure appeared to result in a marked reduction in absenteeism and tardiness.

Time off from work also was used to reinforce data collection with institutional staff early in the program, when staff were asked to collect toilet data on nineteen residents with little success. After several weeks, staff then collected data for five days (baseline) and at this point, were told that data collection for the next five days would be reinforced with half a day off from work for the outstanding data collector in each of three training groups and for the shift training supervisor whose shift collected the most data. After the five-day period, the reinforcement contingency was removed. Thus, a noncontingent-contingent-noncontingent reinforcement experimental design, where each subject served as his own control, was used to assess the staff reinforcement contingency. Results of the study are summarized in Figure IV-8. Contingent reinforcement was correlated with a rather substantial increase in data collection. After the contingency was removed, data collection performance deteriorated. When a follow-up evaluation was made of data collection three months later, the frequency was back to where it had been prior to the introduction of the contingency. Since staff members were given attention weekly for other program

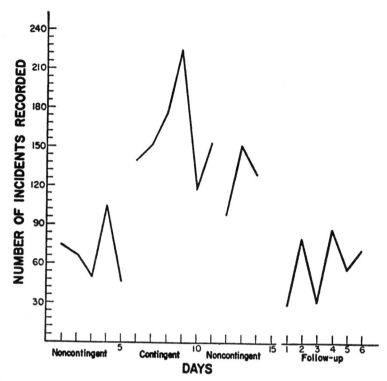

Figure IV-8.   Influence of contingent reinforcement upon data collection by staff.

activities, before and after introduction of the time-off-from-work contingency, these results did not appear to be due to added attention alone (the "Hawthorne Effect").

Following this study, reinforcement was made contingent upon day-to-day data collection, and the problem was eliminated. Each time a supervisor came over to see what a trainer was doing, she began by asking to see the data and provided recognition for data sheets that were properly filled out and that showed residents were making progress in the program.

We also used a number of reinforcements with extra project staff at Columbus State Institute to insure support of our project. We provided the institution with visibility in an effort to reinforce the superintendent. We obtained favorable television and newspaper coverage several times a year. We provided public programs involving the superintendent that reflected favorably on him and on the institution. For example, we held at least one behavior modification workshop each year, and we had tours of our project wards by high level mental health officials from the state central office. The superintendent and clinical director were included in these events.

Each significant staff member in the institution had a behavior modification project staff member assigned to determine his relevant areas of deprivation and provide him with reinforcement in an effort to make him more cooperative. For example, one member of the behavior modification staff found that clinical director had a great interest in the Foster Grandparent Program (which was directly under her jurisdiction) and wanted to involve it more intimately in meaningful institutional activities. So, the behavior modification staff member suggested that Foster Grandparents be used to deal with certain residents who seemed to be significant behavior problems primarily because they were deprived of attention. The clinical director liked this idea, and a particular young educable retarded woman was selected because she had a history of assault on other residents; was slovenly, unmotivated, and uncooperative; and was a general nuisance with the staff on the ward. She was always asking when some member of her family was going to visit her. No one ever recalled her having even one visitor since she had been in the institution—a period greater than ten years. Since she seemed to be particularly attracted to men, a Foster Grandfather was asked to be her "Grandpa." One morning, Mary (a fictitious name) was told her Grandpa had come to visit. She was in her usual state of undress and uncooperativeness. But when she heard she had a visitor, she put on a bra and a clean dress and combed her hair, and then she went out to the reception room to meet her Grandpa. He saw her and told her hello as he gave her a warm smile, and she threw her arms around his neck and gave him a hug as she exclaimed, "Grandpa!" She accepted him without any questions, and he began making two visits a day to see her, once in the morning and once in the afternoon.

His usual routine was to take Mary and go to another building where there was an unused room. There he would have her cut pictures from magazines that could be used in the institutional academic program. He gave her a penny for each picture she cut out (usually 10-15). At the end of this period, he took her to the institutional commissary where she could spend her money on soft drinks or candy and sit in a booth with him and talk. She seemed to enjoy this activity very much. Then when problems arose, such as Mary hitting or biting another resident, Grandpa was so informed by the ward staff, and he would tell Mary he could not take her on an outing if she behaved like that. Thus, a contingent ritual began. When he came to get her, he would always ask the attendant on duty (in Mary's presence) if she had been good. If the attendant said yes, he would smile, say he was proud of her, and give her a pat or hug, and they would go on their outing. But if the attendant said no, he would inquire as to what she had done. Then he would look at her, frown, and say he was very disappointed, hoped she would not do it again, and would not be able to take her on the scheduled outing. But he reassured her that he would return in the afternoon (if he was cancelling the morning visit) or the next morning (if he was cancelling the afternoon visit). He also refused to take her off the ward if she was not wearing a bra (which she routinely rejected), or had on a soiled or torn dress, or was not neat and clean. In this case, he would tell her to go "get cleaned up," and he would wait for her. When she returned, he would inspect her appropriately and comment on how nice she looked, and they would leave to go on the outing. There was a dramatic change for the better in Mary's appearance and behavior. The clinical director seemed to be pleased with this mini-program and began to see some genuine merit to behavior modification.

A second example of reinforcing institutional executive staff to be cooperative involved the hospital administrator and a very attractive RN on the behavior modification project. He obviously was quite taken with her, so she was assigned to accelerate his cooperative behavior. He visited her frequently to talk and periodically invited her for lunch in the institutional cafeteria. She graciously provided him with her company, and from time to time appropriately requested materials and supplies needed to operate the project. Although our data was scanty, she seemed to be an effective social reinforcement for this particular person.

The same general technique was used to gain and maintain the cooperation of the maintenance staff at the institution. Getting maintenance done seemed to be based more on politics than submitting work order requests, and the behavior modification program was greatly dependent upon their support. So, any time any maintenance man came over to the behavior modification ward, he was offered coffee and donuts plus conversation from one of the more attractive female behavior modification staff members. From that point on, there were no more problems with getting burned out lights replaced, leaky faucets repaired, or plugged toilets unplugged.

Finally, a variety of reinforcements were provided to the director of nursing, who controlled all ward staff assignments. She was provided with behavior modification staff to teach nursing education courses, e.g. mental hygiene, and we obtained a grant which supplied the nursing department with a badly needed secretarial position and clerical equipment. We also helped to arrange (and provided funds for) in-service training graduation exercises that brought in high-level state officials and congressmen—a source of recognition for the institution. The director of nursing and the superintendent always were involved in these graduation exercises.

It is important, of course, that those staff members receiving the reinforcement do not interpret it as a bribe or as an exploitive-manipulative act. For this reason, the type of reinforcement and manner in which it is given should be appropriate for the person to whom it is given and should be extended for legitimate, acceptable reasons—acceptable in terms of the mores and values of the person receiving the reinforcement and the community in which the program is taking place.

Just before the conclusion of our behavior modification program at Columbus State Institute, an assessment was made of staff reinforcement preferences in order to better determine what to use for reinforcing different types of staff members associated with the program. These preferences are summarized in Table

IV-IV. The highs and lows for each group are underlined. For example, most administrators preferred extra salary (78%) and only 19 percent preferred recreation at the institution's expense.

SUMMARY

This chapter has been concerned with a system for providing reinforcement to staff involved, either directly or peripherally, with behavior modification programs. It was pointed out that problems arising from insufficient staff reinforcement probably make a significant contribution to lack of success in behavior modification programs. In order to develop an effective, reliable

TABLE IV-IV

REINFORCEMENT PREFERENCES OF STAFF AT
COLUMBUS STATE INSTITUTE
(Calculated in %)

	Group No. 1 %	Group No. 2 %	Group No. 3 %	Group No. 4 %	Group No. 5 %	Group No. 6 %
1. Extra Salary	78	35	91	84	50	72
2. More time off	37	12	36	71	28	13
3. Recognition	22	47	38	21	21	30
4. Letter of commendation	45	35	38	31	21	38
5. Newspaper article	59	18	31	15	21	26
6. Nice break room	41	11	25	53	7	37
7. Special uniform	21	11	7	15	7	34
8. Participate in policy planning	45	11	29	21	57	22
9. Recreational activities at institute's expense	19	11	18	31	7	33
10. Nice office etc.	54	11	33	53	21	22
11. Promotion	45	11	29	37	28	48
12. Challenge	57	23	50	34	28	28
13. Feel qualified to work with mentally retarded	43	17	20	37	21	46
14. Associated with bright people	43	11	27	9	14	34
15. Subordinate's enthusiasm	43	0	3	9	21	16

Group No. 1: Administrators (superintendent, executive staff, supervisors, psychologists, section heads)
Group No. 2: Nurses
Group No. 3: Teachers, activity therapists, speech therapists
Group No. 4: Attendants
Group No. 5: Social workers
Group No. 6: Supportive staff (food service, housekeeping, maintenance, laundry, switchboard, security, storeroom)

staff reinforcement procedure, it frequently may be necessary to provide a system that will support an effective staff reinforcement program. Such a system will require a compatible administrative structure, an effective and economical data or feedback system, and an in-service training program that will teach staff the skills needed to carry out their assigned duties correctly. Three major types of staff reinforcement considered were money, time off from work, and recognition. It was pointed out that recognition can be used in any type of bureaucratic structure even though there are limitations to administrative situations that will permit using money and time off as staff contingent reinforcement.

REFERENCES

Gardner, J. M.; Brust, D., and Watson, L. S.: A scale to measure skill in applying behavior modification techniques to the mentally retarded. *Am J Ment Defic, 4*:633, 1970.

Kugel, L., and Wolfensberger, W.: *Changing Patterns in Residential Services for the Mentally Retarded.* Washington, D.C., President's Committee on Mental Retardation, 1969.

Ullman, L. P., and Krasner, L.: *Case Studies in Behavior Modification.* New York, HR&W, 1965.

Watson, L. S.: *How to Use Behavior Modification with Mentally Retarded and Autistic Children: Programs for Administrators, Teachers, Parents and Nurses.* Libertyville, Behavior Modification Technology, 1972a.

Watson, L. S.: *Teaching Self-help Skills to Children with Behavioral Disorders* (videotape or 16mm film). Libertyville, Behavior Modification Technology, 1972b.

Watson, L. S.: *Teaching Language Skills to Children with Behavioral Disorders* (videotape or 16mm film). Libertyville, Behavior Modification Technology, 1972c.

Watson, L. S.: *Teaching Social-Recreational Skills to Children with Behavioral Disorders* (videotape or 16mm film). Libertyville, Behavior Modification Technology, 1972d.

Watson, L. S.: *Child Behavior Modification: A Manual for Teachers, Nurses and Parents.* New York, Pergamon, 1973.

Watson, L. C.: *Training Proficiency Scale.* Libertyville, Behavior Modification Technology, 1974.

Watson, L. S., and Bassinger, J. F.: Parent training technology: A potential service delivery system. *Ment Retard* (in press).

Watson, L. S.; Gardner, J. F., and Sanders, C.: Shaping and maintaining behavior modification skills in staff members in an MR institution: Columbus State Institute behavior modification program. *Ment Retard*, 9:34, 1971.

Chapter V

INDIVIDUALIZED TREATMENT USING TOKEN ECONOMY METHODS*

Roger L. Patterson, Ph.D.

In 1974, TOKEN economies for psychiatric patients, like so many treatment modalities, may have become burdened by their histories. As Atthowe (1973) has pointed out, most such token economy programs began in large mental hospital wards for regressed chronic patients for the probable reason that nothing was going to do this kind of patient any good anyway. However, in the years since the first token economy systems were developed (Atthowe and Krasner, 1968; Ayllon and Azrin, 1968; Shaefer and Martin, 1969), this method of treatment has been demonstrated to be effective in a wide variety of settings (see Kazdin and Bootzin, 1972, for a recent review). Nevertheless, much of the literature about psychiatric token economy treatment still relates to the same population and the same types of behaviors as were treated in the first published systems. Recent changes in psychiatric treatment indicate that it is time to think of new applications for this methodology.

The trend in modern treatment for psychiatric populations is not to place them in large state institutions, but rather to treat them in smaller facilities close to home (see "The Dean Approach" in Brodsky, 1973). In such facilities, one will be less likely to find large groups of patients with gross deficits of very similar

---

* The work reported in this paper was conducted at Camarillo State Hospital, California and the Mental Health Center of Escambia County, Florida. The conclusions and opinions stated herein are those of the author and should not be construed as official policy of these agencies.

types. It is the thesis of this paper that the implementation of the token economy must be somewhat different with smaller groups of patients with widely differing behavioral problems. The major difference is in the individualization of treatment programs which must be accomplished.

Some examples may help make the point. In a typical back ward of a large institution, one finds large numbers of individuals who dress poorly, do not bathe properly, socialize very little, and do little in the way of ward chores. With such cases, it is relatively easy to identify general categories of behavior which need to be produced and/or increased for most of the population. Such items as tobacco, candy, and desserts may also function as effective and readily available reinforcers for most of this group.

In contrast, consider a small psychiatric ward or day-treatment center in which may be found such people as an intelligent, well-groomed young man of nineteen who engages in bizarre stealing; a profoundly retarded man of thirty-nine who is kept locked up primarily because he hugs people on the street; a kindly, well-groomed, hardworking lady of sixty who speaks utter absurdities about herself and her family; a twenty-nine-year-old man who dresses slovenly, constantly insults people, refuses to do any work, and whose conversation sounds like a recording of an encyclopedia.

It has been adequately demonstrated that token systems provide a useful means of systematically applying appropriate contingencies to modify a vast number of behaviors (Kazdin and Bootzin, 1972). It is now also widely recognized that a variety of other behavior therapy techniques in addition to contingency management are useful in changing behavior (Franks, 1969). Therefore, a comprehensive treatment center which seeks to treat a large variety of behavioral problems should make use of as many of these behavioral change methods as is necessary in each case. This means that token economy methods may be used both as a method of directly altering targeted responses, or in combination with other treatment methods. The latter combination can be a most powerful means of changing many behaviors. It is this type of treatment combination, referred to here as the individualized token economy (T.E.), which will be discussed in this paper.

The application of complete behavioral programs in such a precise way almost always involves the development of a behavioral prescription for the individual. The operations involved in applying individual behavioral prescriptions of many types may be performed by a variety of paraprofessionals with adequate professional supervision (Ayllon and Azrin, 1968; Tharpe and Wetzel, 1969). However, it has been the experience of the author that the operation of a facility in which a number of behavioral prescriptions are simultaneously in progress and are being applied by means of the cooperative effort of several professionals and paraprofessionals in one treatment unit requires that all efforts be coordinated by one person. In this paper, such a person will be referred to as the program director. The tasks of the program director in developing the individualized T.E. include those of acquiring and training a staff and creating a *system* of application which will ensure that the most effective individual programs will be devised and properly implemented.

The problem of staff acquisition in mental institutions has, in the past, been all too simple: The nursing supervisor handled it by assigning various nursing personnel to a particular ward. (In those cases in which the program director had university connections and/or grant money, he usually obtained the services of college students.) The predominant use of nursing personnel in behavioral programs is a direct descendant of the dominance of the medical model. The contributions of many of these personnel have been admirable (Liberman, et al., 1973; Sibbach, 1969). Also, it is indisputable that adequate medical care utilizing nursing personnel is necessary for the population being discussed. A sufficient number of members of the nursing staff must be available to meet needs of the population. However, it is not necessarily true that nursing personnel will have had the best training or the greatest interest in working with behavioral programs. The movement of treatment to specially developed localized facilities will hopefully produce an improved system of employee selection. Such treatment centers should be relatively free from a long tradition of domination by nursing organizational hierarchies.

There is a sizeable body of potential employees available who have the interest and the training in basic behavioral science to make good behavioral technicians: the people with subdoctoral degrees in psychology. Consider the logic of employing a person with a B.A. or M.A. in psychology in this capacity. He or she will, in almost all instances, have had introductory courses in learning theory, experimental psychology, statistics and measurement, abnormal psychology, and others, in addition to all the training that is necessary for a liberal arts degree. Besides this background knowledge, the person with a degree in psychology will have demonstrated a primary interest in the sciences of behavior. Tharpe and Wetzel (1969) have documented the success of such personnel in implementing behavior change programs.

The specialized training of personnel is discussed at length elsewhere in this book (see especially papers by Kazdin and McInnis); so it will not be pursued in this chapter. There is a point which this author wishes to emphasize here: Training is a *continuous* process. It is the author's experience that some innovation which must be taught to the staff is required with many patients. Also, behavioral methodology is constantly being modified and developed. The program director in all cases must take the responsibiilty of seeing that appropriate innovations are applied. This requires constant staff training.

The development of a system of individualized behavioral prescriptions and application involves primarily the following components:

1. a method of rapid and effective individual prescription development,
2. the communication of these prescriptions to all relevant personnel,
3. the collection of highly diversified but reliable individual data,
4. frequent and rapid behavioral prescription revision, and
5. a method of assuring that all staff carry out the prescriptions properly and collect the required data. The program director must, with the advice and cooperation of his staff, develop efficient routines for the performance of these duties.

The author has served as program director in two widely differing individualized T.E.'s. One was the Clinical Research Unit (CRU) at Camarillo State Hospital, California (Liberman, et al., 1973). The other was the Day Treatment Program (DTP) of the Community Mental Health Center of Escambia County, Florida. Both of these programs were individualized because of the diversity of behavioral problems dealt with in each. The systems employed in these two behavioral change centers will be described below. No claims are made that these methods are in any way ideal. The only purpose in describing these programs is to present the reader with two examples of individualized T.E. programs which were found to be workable.

CLINICAL RESEARCH UNIT*

The first program to be described was developed on the Clinical Research Unit (CRU) of Camarillo State Hospital in California.† This token economy program did not start out with the intent of complete individualization. Rather, the program began with the posting of a list of ward jobs with accompanying payments and a prominently displayed list of reinforcers with the costs.‡ However, we found ourselves forced to move rapidly in the direction of increased individualization. In order to understand why this was so, it will be helpful to describe the CRU and its functions.

The CRU is a twelve-bed ward in a large state hospital. Its purpose, stated most simply, is to conduct research on a wide variety of patient types in order to develop more effective means of modifying their behavior, and to disseminate these treatment methods throughout the hospital and the state and to interested professionals in general by means of professional publications.

---

* The Clinical Research Unit was begun by Dr. Robert Liberman who continued to be involved in all activities on this unit. James Teigen, M.S.W., also assisted in most of the work.

† The interpretations and conclusions in this section of the paper are those of the author and are not to be construed as official or necessarily reflecting the policy of the California Department of Mental Hygiene.

‡ Dr. Robert Grippe, then a psychology intern, and Ms. Gina Manchester, a psychiatric technician, did much of the beginning work on this program.

The nursing staff to provide total twenty-four-hour coverage usually consisted of about seven registered nurses and seven psychiatric technicians. These people were selected primarily because of their interest in participating in this type of program. After selection, they were trained in methods of behavior modification and data collection. The professional staff consisted of a psychiatrist, a clinical psychologist (who was named program director), a social worker, and a research assistant.

The reason for the need for individualization came from the mission of the CRU to develop methods for a wide variety of patients. The population of state hospitals does not consist exclusively of those who are usually described as "chronic, backward, regressed patients" who lack grooming and self-care skills or who refuse to interact with others. People with a great variety of problems come to such places for a number of reasons. Accordingly, after several months of operation we found ourselves with some people who were perhaps overcompulsive and too compliant about grooming and ward jobs. (In fact, the opportunity to groom himself was used as a reinforcer with one man.) Some patients had good social skills, or socialized too much. At the same time we had some patients who were deficient in these areas or who had problems unrelated to any of these. Under these conditions, the posted lists of reinforcers and jobs made less and less sense.

The system which we developed for specifying each individual's program of behavior therapy involved standardized forms for token management systems, and especially written prescriptions with accompanying data sheets for programs which did not fit the standard forms or which did not involve tokens. (Standard forms simplify and systematize, but treatment should not be bound by their use.) The standard form for the token program appears in Figure V-1.

It contains spaces for specifying which behaviors were to be consequated, and the consequence for each (the payment or charge). The form also included enough spaces to record on a daily basis whether or not the consequence was administered for a total period of two weeks. Note that such a format requires that a new sheet be made, and thus that the program be updated

TOKEN ECONOMY TARGET BEHAVIOR REVIEW FORM

Patient _____   Therapists _____   _____

TARGET BEHAVIORS FOR COMING WEEK: Based on Previous Assessment.

Item   Token Amount & Schedule

1._____   1._____
  _____   _____

2._____   2._____
  _____   _____

3._____   3._____
  _____   _____

4._____   4._____
  _____   _____

5._____   5._____
  _____   _____

6._____   6._____
  _____   _____

7._____   7._____
  _____   _____

ASSESSMENT: Check whether above items were completed. Use zero (O) if item not completed.

Dates_____thru_____	M	Tu	W	Th	F	S	S	M	Tu	W	Th	F	S	S	
1.															1.
2.															2.
3.															3.
4.															4.
5.															5.
6.															6.
7.															7.

SUGGESTED NEW GOALS: Base goals on your assessment. Be specific about behaviors & reinforcement to be used in attaining new target behavior. Add comments about the quality of the previous weeks behavior. Be specific about which link in a reverse chaining procedure the patient is at.

_____
_____
_____
_____
_____
_____
_____
_____
_____
_____
_____
_____
_____
_____

Figure V-1.   Data sheet for the CRU.

at least every two weeks, although program changes could be
made at any time. The form lends itself to regular and rapid
update not only bcause it contains spaces for no more than two
weeks of data, but also because the behavior consequated,

the frequency of performance, and the consequence used are displayed on one sheet. The sheet also contains space at the bottom for nursing staff members to recommend program changes.

The way that programs were initiated involved the combined use of referral data, interview data obtained from the patient and others concerned, behavioral observations, and suggestions by *anyone* working on the ward. However, the initial observations were not left to chance. When a new patient came to the ward he was assigned primary therapists on the morning and atfernoon shifts who had the responsibility of making initial program suggestions. These primary therapists, or designated substitutes, had the task of assuring that their patients' treatment was properly conducted throughout their stay at the CRU. This author, as program director, had the final authority of issuing all program instructions regardless of whose idea may have been incorporated into the final prescription. This was found by experience to be necessary to avoid the confusion arising from information coming from too many sources. The initial token programs were generally issued after week's observation. The final token program was usually kept on a clipboard in the nurses' station, convenient to all.

When a token program was revised, usually at the end of a two-week period, the primary therapist was again required to gather comments from the other staff members and to recommend program changes (if the therapist's off-days fell at the end of the program period, he or she was to fill out the form earlier or to instruct his or her relief). Recommended changes were written in the space provided on the bottom of the data sheet. The director, the social worker, and the research assistant wrote new programs based on the recorded performance data and the suggestions. These were issued after final approval of the director.

It may have been noted by the reader that although the data-recording method described above provided performance and token payment data, it did not provide token spending data which is necessary to keep a client's economy balanced. A very simple system to accomplish this task was suggested by Dr. Robert Liberman, the CRU psychiatrist. This method involved the use of a token box with two compartments for each client. The client's name and the code number with which his tokens were marked were attached to these two compartments. (Code numbers were used to ensure that each client received and spent only his own tokens.) One compartment was filled with a recorded number of tokens before the client arose each morning. He was then paid with the tokens from this compartment as he earned them during the day. The other compartment was used to deposit the tokens as he spent them. It was, therefore, a simple matter for the night shift to count the number of tokens remaining in the pay-out box and subtract them from the amount placed in that box the night before to determine a client's earnings that day (this same amount was, of course, separately recorded on his program sheet). The number of tokens spent by each patient (in the paid-in box) was similarly recorded each day along with the daily balance. With these data, it was a very simple matter to operate a "bank" and to adjust payments so that clients became neither too rich nor too poor. These data were consulted in order to determine appropriate payments and costs to attach to various behaviors for which token contingencies were required. It should be noted here that token economies which use token response costs or "fines" must be very carefully administered to avoid debts. Subjects who go into debt frequently lose almost all positive motivation (Doty, et al., 1974).

Some illustrative examples will be useful to show how it was possible to tailor token payments to individual needs by means of this system. In the case of the sixty-year-old, hardworking, well-groomed, sociable lady* who spoke absurdities about herself and her family, it was decided to make *all* her token earnings dependent upon her giving truthful answers to questions about herself and her family. This procedure proved effective (Patterson and Teigen, 1973).

Another example is that of a young man who made very unusual grabbing motions with his hands while staring off into space. When asked what he was doing at such times, he reported that he was seeing girls and trying to grab them. Observations

---

* This lady had already undergone considerable treatment by means of behavior modification as described by Liberman, et al., 1973.

of his token earnings and spendings indicated that he would spend a large number of tokens for a variety of reinforcers and that he could be kept active by means of token-reinforced tasks. He was, therefore, kept as active as feasible. The token-reinforced activity did not eliminate the undesired behavior, so it was decided to attempt to reduce the grabbing motions directly by treating them by the behavior therapy method frequently known as negative practice (Yates, 1958). Tokens assisted in the accomplishment of this method of therapy by paying this subject for performing his practice sessions and also for participating in separate data collection sessions, in addition to paying him for remaining active. (Both the treatment and data gathering were very boring for the subject.) The behavior was found to be almost totally eliminated after treatment, although it returned at a very low frequency after about two months without negative practice sessions (Patterson, unpublished manuscript).

In contrast to the above two cases, the method of token payment solely for the performance of ward tasks was used in the case of an overly aggressive, obese young woman of borderline intelligence. This woman said that she wanted to become a housekeeper. However, referral data and baseline observations indicated that her personal grooming and housekeeping skills definitely needed improvement. Based on this information, she was assigned large numbers of ward chores to fill her working day. She was paid tokens for maintaining her grooming and for performing the tasks at a level which should be required of a professional housekeeper.

The above three examples represent extremes from the payment of all tokens earned for a single desired behavior, to a mixture of different types of behavior, to the payment of all tokens for chores and grooming. In addition to those on this continuum, there were patients on the CRU who received no tokens at all. These patients were those who were being treated by other behavior therapy methods and who participated willingly in all required behavior without the necessity of reinforcement beyond normal social amenities. Creating token programs for such patients would have been wasted effort.

The token programs using the standard form were relatively

easy to revise, communicate, and store. Old token programs were kept in individual patient notebooks after they were removed from the clipboard and served as permanent data sources. However, special token programs or other behavior therapy programs which did not involve tokens (both of these were called special programs) were harder to communicate.

A memo system was devised to facilitate such communication. A data room next to the nurse's station contained individual mailboxes for each member of the staff, including the janitor. Any time that a special program was initiated (most of our clients had from one to three of these) or changed, everyone received a memo from the director containing exact instructions for performing the program operations and collecting the data. A sample data sheet was included. Each staff member kept a personal file in a filing cabinet in the nursing station for storage and ready reference to all programs. One copy of each special program was also placed in each client's notebook and on the program clipboard. In addition, all new programs were posted in a space reserved for this purpose on a large bulletin board in the nurses' station. Such redundant distribution of these memos assured that all staff members were informed in written form of all special programs.

The system did not rely exclusively on memos for communication, however. The method of shift change in this hospital allowed for a half-hour overlap of the shifts at each change. Information could thus be transmitted verbally from the A.M. to the P.M. to the night shifts, and from nights back to the A.M. shift. The program director or one of the professional staff was almost always present at the afternoon change-of-shift meeting. At this time, program changes could be explained, demonstrated, or modeled as necessary to the two shifts primarily responsible for the programs. This actually constituted almost constant in-service training. In addition to these half-hour meetings, a one-hour change-of-shift meeting was scheduled for A.M.'s and P.M.'s twice weekly. The night shift and the A.M. shift met together with the professional staff once weekly. The longer meetings permitted additional time for training, working with personnel problems, and other types of communication.

All of these meetings also provided an opportunity for a different function, feedback, and social reinforcement of staff. An attempt was made by the director to open each meeting by having either himself, or preferably, members of the nursing staff, give any new successful data available. The members of the staff who were primarily responsible for the successes were given full credit. This procedure combined knowledge of success with recognition for achievement, both of which have been used as human reinforcers (Skinner, 1968). It was only after such success presentations that problems were dealt with. In the experience of the author, staff meetings frequently become sessions emphasizing failure rather than serving the purpose of emphasizing success. For some reason, treatment teams seem to have a tendency to spend a great deal of time talking about failures and problems. It is the opinion of this author that reversing this emphasis serves to greatly boost staff morale and to improve performance.

Feedback and social reinforcement for appropriate staff behavior were not restricted to staff meetings. Individuals were socially reinforced on an individual basis, and discussions about the progress of individual clients were held with individuals, whenever possible. The CRU also published a newsheet on a weekly or biweekly basis which gave progress reports on all clients, as well as information about staff, publications, etc. The newssheet ended with a humor section to which staff members contributed jokes, usually about each other (Patterson, et al., 1972).

DAY TREATMENT PROGRAM

The individualization in the T.E. program of the DTP of the Mental Health Center in Escambia County, Pensacola, Florida, accomplished many of the same purposes as those described above. However, the T.E. *system* differed considerably.*

The DTP was divided into an adolescent and an adult program. Although each day's regularly planned group activities were always *available,* they were never required of anyone who

---

* The method of recording daily activities and token payments in the Day Treatment Program was developed under the leadership of Rex Haire, Ph.D.

could use a different activity at that time (so long as someone was available to assist in the alternative activity). However, individualization of assignments took place primarily *within* the scheduled activities.

The DTP staff consisted of the director (the author); six therapists, each with a baccalaureate or master's degree in nursing or social science; a home economics supervisor; and a teacher trained to work with the disturbed. Each therapist had up to five clients assigned to him. Two of the therapists and the teacher worked only with adolescent clients.

Treatment planning for each new client began with a staff intake interview. Someone, usually the director, summarized relevant data from known history and the referral source at the beginning of each interview. The client, and sometimes family members, were then given a behaviorally focused interview in which questions were asked by the staff in an attempt to define needed behavioral changes. After the intake, each new client was assigned a therapist. This therapist had the responsibility of defining a set of goals for behavioral change for his client by the end of one week in the program. Goal Attainment Scaling (GAS; Kiresuk and Sherman, 1968) was used as a method of defining behavioral goals for each client and measuring his progress in the program.

The GAS method was devised to measure long-term outcome of treatment programs in mental health centers. The level of outcome of treatment expected by a certain date for each goal is defined in a measureable way, and from two to four other possible levels of outcome for each goal are similarly defined. The rule is that there must be at least one possible outcome defined at a level more favorable than the expected, and one level similarly defined which is less favorable than the expected. This procedure creates a measurement scale which can be used to evaluate treatment progress at a specified time.

In addition to the intake interview, several other sources of data were used to define goals and to develop prescriptions. Individual meetings were held with the primary therapist as needed. Reports of observed behavior in the DTP were obtained. The program also included a "Problem Definition Group" held daily for all new clients for their first one or two weeks in the program. This group sought to teach new clients to define their own difficulties in terms of behavior they themselves needed to change. Although considerable effort was made to discover and define all goals shortly after the client entered the program, new goals could be defined at any time.

The therapists and the teacher met weekly with the director on an individual basis to confer about new patient goals, to review progress data on previously developed goals, and to develop individual behavioral programs to achieve newly defined goals. In the DTP, such meetings could be held on an individual basis with each staff member each week, since everyone was there at the same time. This offers distinct advantages over the hospital situation, where it is impossible to meet with everyone individually on a frequent basis. Staff meetings, in addition to the intake interviews, were held twice weekly. These served much the same purpose as those described in the hospital setting.

By means of these individual and group staff meetings, the director was automatically involved in all treatment plans and informed about client progress. He could therefore indirectly monitor staff behavior. This procedure also allowed the director to make sure that all procedures were being followed. An attempt was made by the director to turn these meetings into success feedback and social reinforcement sessions. Staff were encouraged to initiate each meeting with reports of successful clients. The director responded by immediately recognizing these successes and praising staff for their good performance.

The individual programs involved the use of daily scheduled group activities as well as activities designed only for specific clients. A major group activity was called "Behavior Rehearsal Group." In this group clients rehearsed specific types of social behaviors which they needed to learn or to improve upon by role playing. The role-playing scenes were videotaped and immediately played back to the entire group. The group was encouraged to make comments directed towards specifying behaviors which showed improvement and which needed to be further improved. Tokens were given on an individualized basis for a variety of behaviors in this group. Clients could be paid for merely coming to the group, for commenting about others' performance, for engaging in role playing, or for having successfully role-played behaviors that they themselves needed to learn. Clients actually engaging in role playing could also be paid for successfully specifying components of their own behavior which had changed or which needed changing. Of course, the ultimate outcome of behavior rehearsal was the performance of the actual behavior in the real environment (this was possible in the DTP whereas it might not be in an institution). Clients could obviously be paid off for achievement of this step.

Another standard group was called "Interpersonal Group." This activity required clients to make certain types of statements to each other according to the rules of several sensitivity games.*

The purpose was to teach clients to relate to each other in various types of ways using both verbal and nonverbal cues. The procedure also required clients to correctly identify the interpersonal communications they were receiving. Again, clients were paid tokens on an individual basis according to the particular types of these behaviors they needed to improve upon.

Other therapy groups used in the DTP found little use for tokens. These included a "Rational Emotive Group" (Ellis, 1962) and a form of desensitization based on the methods of Wolpe and Lazarus (1966), and Richardson and Suinn (1973), modified by the director to be useful for groups of individuals with *different* sources of anxiety (Patterson, unpublished manuscript).

Tokens were found to be very useful in the adolescent classroom. The adolescent clients in this setting varied tremendously in their level of achievement (from pre-first-grade to college freshman). They also varied a great deal in their classroom behaviors. For these reasons, program individualization was quite essential here. As examples, some clients were paid for sitting in their desks while attending to a book for a few minutes, others were paid for completing grade-level assignments, some were paid only for asking appropriate questions about assignments, and one very compulsive boy was actually paid for leaving his work long enough to take a ten-minute break.

---

* These were obtained from Psychology Today Games, P.O. Box 60278, Terminal Annex, Los Angeles, California 90060.

Other activities in the DTP which provided considerable opportunity for individualized payments included shop, meal preparation, art, sports, grooming, learning about other clients, etc. Since DTP was actually located in the community, token payments could be made for activities outside the mental health center. For example, adolescent clients were typically paid tokens for their performance in a few classes in a community school before they were taken off the token program. Adults returning from mental institutions (and others) were sometimes paid for riding city buses, attending community social events (church was a favorite), driving a car, and many other ordinary daily activities.

With the brief program outline as background, the system can now be explained whereby all this individualization was achieved. A daily activities form was made out for each client by his primary therapist when he reported each day. This was done at a meeting of each therapist with his clients. This form, a sample of which appears in Figure V-2, included a space for each activity in which he was to participate along with the scheduled time, and the specific behavior for which he was to be paid or charged during each activity. Spaces were included to indicate the payment given to, or charges paid by, the client beside each assignment. There were also spaces for making behavioral counts and any needed comments. The client was given one copy of this sheet and another was placed on a clipboard for the observer to keep.

The actual observations and counts of the various individual behaviors were made by an observer who had one of the clipboards with the daily assignments sheets for the group he was scheduled to observe. These observers were usually volunteers who were given brief training in behavioral observations and counting. (A former therapist who desired part-time work was hired to recruit, train, and supervise volunteers.) Many of the volunteers were undergraduate or graduate psychology students from several universities. Others were ex-clients and housewives not otherwise employed. The staff leader of the particular activity had to see that appropriate observations were made as part of his duty in this activity.

DAILY SCHEDULE

Client _____   Therapist _____   Date

Special Instructions _____

ACTIVITY	TOKENS		COMMENTS
	Pay	Charge	
8:30 - 9:00 Planning Meeting			
9:00 - 9:30 Behavior Rehearsal			Pay 2 tokens for each comment about another's rehearsal. Charge 5 for each inappropriate laugh.
9:30 - 10:00			
10:00 - 10:30			
10:30 - 11:00 Canteen & Socialization			Pay 5 if he converses for 10 minutes.
11:30 - 12:00 Meal Preparation			Pay 10 for setting tables
12:00 - 12:30 Lunch			Charge 30
12:30 - 1:00 Play checkers with Mrs. M.			Pay 10
1:00 - 1:30 Interpersonal Group			Pay 2 for each 10 minutes of participation
1:30 - 2:00			
2:00 - 2:30			
2:30 - 3:00 Canteen & Socialization			Pay 5 for 10 minute conversation
3:00 - 3:30 Evaluation Meeting			

Comments: _____

Figure V-2.   Data sheet for the DTP.

An accounting period was the last activity of each day. During this period, the earnings and expenditures of each client (taken from the program sheet) were tallied by his therapist and any balance remaining was entered into a bank account. Another function of this period of the day was to remind the clients of their accomplishments and areas in which they needed to improve.

Backup reinforcers for the tokens included lunch, coffee, canteen items, trading stamps, telephone privileges, time with a favored therapist, and items supplied by families and other interested individuals. A somewhat unusual source of reinforcers consisted of items supplied by the vocational rehabilitation service for clients who were sponsored by that agency. These might consist of articles of clothing, tools, taxi chits, opportunities to attend classes, or any other vocationally related items. This latter type of reinforcer was especially valuable for higher level clients.

The system described above for prescribing the behavior to be reinforced for each of several activities sounds very complicated. Indeed, it could be so in its extreme form. However, the prescription for many clients was greatly simplified because it was frequently possible to define a class of behaviors which could be reinforced in more than one activity. For example, several clients had the problem of talking about matters which were totally irrelevant to the activity going on around them. In such cases, it was possible to reinforce the clients with tokens and praise for making relevant statements, regardless of the activity. Ignoring the irrelevant statements or fines could be the consequence for the undesirable behavior. Other clients had problems in making interpersonal statements to others, or in maintaining eye contact while speaking. The Behavior Rehearsal and Interpersonal Groups were especially valuable for correcting such behaviors, but these persons could be reinforced when these behaviors occurred in any activity. Individual shaping sessions with a therapist or volunteer were arranged in addition to group sessions for persons with many kinds of problems. Completing any activity was difficult for some clients. For these people, payoff was simply based on the completion of each activity.

The case of one client is particularly interesting. He had the disturbing behavior of casually insulting people almost every time he spoke to them. The initial therapeutic effort was to reinforce a supposedly incompatible behavior by paying him tokens only for complimenting other people. Part of each behavior rehearsal session was set aside for him to rehearse compliment-giving. He very quickly developed a high rate of delivering phoney-sounding compliments in many activities, but the frequency data revealed that he also maintained a high rate of delivery of insults. The assumption that compliments and insults were incompatible was false. The strategy at this point was then changed so that he was no longer paid for anything. He was simply given a supply of tokens each morning and told that he would be charged one token for each insult. With this latter procedure, his rate of both phoney compliments and insults rapidly decreased and his conversation became more nearly normal.

A special method was employed to eliminate token-mediated reinforcement from a client's life when he was being prepared for discharge. This involved promoting the person to "senior client" status. A senior client was given the privilege of access to all reinforcers without the exchange of tokens. This freedom from tokens seemed to function as a reinforcer based on the comments of the clients and the fact that they were willing to improve their performance on some task(s) or to do additional tasks in order to achieve this status. The clients were also required to maintain their higher level of performance in order to remain senior clients. The tasks required of senior clients were made as relevant to the person's post-discharge needs as possible. For example, these people might be required to ride city buses each day, to practice driving, to go for job interviews, to cook dinner at home each night, or to do a host of other specified duties based on individual need.

At this point it is probably most useful to give a summary of the success of the DTP program using the Goal Attainment data. However, before giving the data it is necessary to explain that we found that two types of GAS data were needed. This is because goals set for attainment while in the treatment program were frequently not the same as the post-discharge goals. The treatment data obtained by the observers in the DTP were in the form of the frequency and/or the quality of observed behaviors (some self-report data was also used). One example given above for one client was frequency of insults.

The post-discharge data frequently consisted of reports from the ex-client, his family and friends, his vocational rehabilitation counselor, etc., concerning the adequacy of his living arrangement, his behavior towards social groups, the degree of job success, etc. To continue with the example of the client who insulted people, some of his post-discharge goals included his willingness to do chores around the house (he was started on a behavioral contract for this purpose while in treatment), allowing his stepfather to watch television without interruption, attending social functions, and others. These data were primarily obtained from his mother.

"Success-during-treatment" data were obtained for a total of ninety-four goals set for thirty-three different clients. (Data could be reported only for those clients who stayed in treatment for the length of time, usually four weeks, set for measuring goal attainment at the time the goals were initially defined.) These data indicate that, on the average, we obtained a level of success slightly greater than the expected.

The follow-up data were usually obtained at periods of one, three, and six months after discharge. The follow-up goals were defined for the level of success expected one month after discharge. Post-discharge data available for forty-three clients* one month after termination of treatment showed that on the average, these clients attained a level almost equal to (slightly above) the expected level of success. The three-month data available for twenty-eight of these clients showed that they generally continued at the level expected for one month after discharged. However, the mean of the six-month data available for sixteen ex-clients indicated that there was a slight improvement over the level expected for one month after discharge.

---

* The seeming incongruity of having more follow-up than treatment data is explained by two factors: We started using GAS to measure long-term outcome *before* we used this method to measure treatment goals; and post-discharge goals were set for some clients who dropped out of treatment before the period of measurement for their treatment goals had been completed.

These data are encouraging in that they show that the individualized T.E. as we used it in the DTP had long-lasting effects.

SUMMARY

At this point rather than to continue with details, it is probably more useful to summarize some of the major objectives of this presentation. The major objective was to show that it is possible to achieve a high degree of individualization in behavior therapy programs involving a number of staff working with a group of clients with very difficult problems. However, considerable thought must go into the development of a system of coordinated procedures to achieve this result. The two such systems which were described functioned in very different settings (a large state hospital and a community mental health center). These were intended to serve only as examples. Although other workers in this field are encouraged to borrow from these examples whatever they may find useful, it is hoped that considerably more work will be done in developing methods for the widespread application of precise behavior modification for that vast group of people most frequently referred to by the general public as the "mentally ill."

REFERENCES

Atthowe, J. M., Jr.: Token economies come of age. *Behav Ther,* 4:646, 1973.

Atthowe, J. M., Jr., and Krasner, L.: Preliminary report on the application of contingent reinforcement procedure (token economy) on a "chronic" psychiatric ward. *J Abnorm Psychol,* 73:37, 1968.

Ayllon, T., and Azrin, N. H.: *The Token Economy: A Motivational System for Therapy and Rehabilitation.* New York, Appleton, 1968.

Brodsky, S. L.: Community alternatives to criminal and juvenile justice processes. In Brodsky, S. L., and Knudten, R. D. (Eds.): *Strategies for Delinquency Prevention in the Schools.* Tuscaloosa, University of Alabama, 1973.

Doty, D. W.; McInnis, Titus, and Paul, G. L.: Remediation of negative side effects of an on-going response-cost system with chronic mental patients. *J Appl Behav Anal,* 7:191, 1974.

Ellis, A.: *Reason and Emotion in Psycho-Therapy.* New York, Lyle Stuart, 1962.

Franks, C. M.: *Behavior Therapy: Appraisal and Status.* New York, McGraw, 1969.

Kazdin, A. E., and Bootzin, R. R.: The token economy: An evaluative review. *J Appl Behav Anal,* 5:343, 1972.

Kiresuk, T. J., and Sherman, R. E.: Goal attainment scaling: A general method for evaluating comprehensive community mental health programs. *Community Ment Health J,* 4:443, 1968.

Liberman, R. P.; Teigen, J. R.; Patterson, R. L., and Baker, V.: Reducing delusional speech in chronic paranoid schizophrenics. *J Appl Behav Anal,* 6:57, 1973.

Patterson, R. L.; Cooke, C., and Liberman, R. P.: Reinforcing the reinforcers: A method of supplying feedback to nursing personnel. *Behav Ther,* 3:444, 1972.

Patterson, R. L., and Teigen, J. R.: Conditioning and post-hospital generalization of nondelusional response in a chronic psychotic patient. *J Appl Behav Anal,* 6:65, 1973.

Richardson, F. C., and Suinn, R. M.: A comparison of tradition, systematic desensitization, accelerated massed desensitization and anxiety management training in the treatment of mathematics anxiety. *Behav Ther,* 4:212, 1973.

Schaefer, H. H., and Martin, P. L.: *Behavioral Therapy.* New York. McGraw, 1969.

Sibbach, L.: Description of the token economy program. In Ball, T. S. (Ed.): *The Establishment and Administration of Operant Conditioning Programs in a State Hospital for the Retarded.* California Mental Health Research Symposium, No. 4, California Department of Mental Hygiene, Sacramento, 1969.

Skinner, B. F.: *The Technology of Teaching.* New York, Appleton, 1968.

Tharpe, R. G., and Wetzel, R. J.: *Behavior Modification in the National Environment.* New York, Acad Pr, 1969.

Wolpe, J., and Lazarus, A. A.: *Behavior Therapy Techniques.* New York, Pergamon, 1966.

Yates, A. J.: The application of learning theory to the treatment of tics. *J Abnorm Soc Psychol,* 56:175, 1958.

THE USE OF A "JOB BOARD" TO SIMPLIFY AND STANDARDIZE A TOKEN ECONOMY

CHARLES J. WALLACE, PH.D.; JOHN R. DAVIS, AND VAL BAKER*

S INCE ITS INCEPTION in November of 1970, the Clinical Research Unit (CRU) at Camarillo State Hospital has used a token economy to modify patient behavioral excesses and deficits. The purpose of this paper is to describe the current token economy which is now rather different than that which was first employed (a description of the initial economy can be found in Patterson's chapter in this book). The CRU is a twelve-bed, coed unit with a staff of fourteen nurses and psychiatric technicians, a psychiatrist, psychologist, social worker, and research assistant.

SYSTEMS OF MODIFYING EXCESSES AND DEFICITS

Before describing the token economy in detail, it is necessary to describe the function and place of the economy in the CRU's systems of modifying behavioral excesses and deficits. Patients are most often referred to the CRU from other units within Camarillo State Hospital for modification of numerous behaviors. Many of these behaviors are the same from patient to patient and are of such a type that their modification is frequently critical to a patient's successful placement in a community facility.

---

* The opinions or conclusions stated in this paper are those of the authors and are not to be construed as official or as necessarily reflecting the policy of the California Department of Health. The authors also appreciate the support and suggestions given by Robert Paul Liberman, M.D.

Standardized systems for the modification of these behaviors have been developed and are routinely applied to all patients. Each system includes a standard definition of appropriate or inappropriate behaviors, a standard consequation procedure, and a standard means of collecting and recording data. Four such standard systems have been implemented to deal with the following four categories of behaviors: eating behaviors, personal hygiene, destructive and assaultive behaviors, and performance of routine self-care and household tasks such as making a bed.

There are, of course, behaviors which do not fit into these standardized systems and which are generally the primary reason for referral. These behaviors vary from patient to patient and may include tics, hysterical coughs, fetishes, delusional speech, etc.; since these behaviors are so different from person to person, a flexible system has been developed in which each patient has an individual treatment program to modify his or her specifically targeted excess or deficit. The program includes a definition of the targeted behavior which is unique to that program, an individualized consequation procedure, and an individualized data collection and recording device.

The staff behaviors required to record and consequate the target behaviors are thoroughly detailed in a dittoed memo which is distributed to all staff members. Each patient has a clipboard which is hung on a pegboard in the nurses' station and which contains that patient's most recent treatment memo and that day's data collection sheet.

The flexibility of the individualized system is best illustrated by the variety of consequation and data collection techniques that may take place in a day. Staff may be asked to observe a patient thirty-six times during the day and note the presence or absence of the targeted behavior during the one-minute observation period, to have four fifteen-minute chats during which delusional speech may be consequated, to interact for thirty-six brief periods with a patient as long as the patient is not self-abusing, to conduct three ten-minute sessions in which eye contact is reinforced on a CRF schedule, to participate in daily assertion training groups, etc.

Thus, the four standardized systems plus the individualized

system allow the CRU both to modify those behaviors which may be wholly unique to the patient under consideration and to shape those behaviors which are essential to every patient's successful living in the community or in the hospital. It is the token economy which functions as the standardized system to shape appropriate performance of routine self-care and household tasks.

THE TOKEN ECONOMY

Job Performance

The CRU's daily chores are divided into ten major routines such as cleaning the dining room, cleaning the dayroom, cleaning the female and male bathrooms, and cleaning the hallways. Some of the ten major routines are repeated throughout the day for a daily total of twenty-three various major routines. The twenty-three routines are composed of 102 jobs such as washing the dining room tables after lunch, emptying the dayroom ashtrays in the afternoon, and mopping and sweeping the male bathroom floor in the evening. The name of each job, the criteria for completion, and the token value are mimeographed on cards measuring 3½ by 5½ inches.

Organization and Display of Jobs

The job cards, segregated by major routine, are placed in chronological order on a job board constructed so that it is similar to the fixtures used to store employee time cards. The board consists of a doubled-over, plastic mattress cover thumb-tacked to a four-by-four-foot piece of particle board. The doubled-over cover has been sewn vertically so that it has five 1½-inch-wide columns. The cover is sewn horizontally into twenty-eight 1½-inch rows. Each column thus has twenty-eight cells that are 1½ inches high by either 6 or 1½ inches wide. The first layer of the plastic cover is slit widthwise to make a slot in which the job cards are placed. The dimensions of the cells are such that the name of each job is always visible with one job card layered in front of and below the preceding card.

The board is placed in the nurses' station so that staff members can quickly see the daily routine. In addition, two sets of 1¼-by-3-inch cards are involved—one set with the specific time periods allotted for each major routine and the other set with patient names. The time period cards are placed in the column to the left of the job cards, while the patient name cards are placed in the slot with the job card corresponding to the job the patient has been assigned. Thus, staff members can see at a glance not only the time at which each routine and its associated jobs are to be performed, but also the patients who have been assigned to the various jobs.

Patient-Carried Records

In the hope of simplifying data collection, the unit of exchange was at one point switched from a token to a "credit." Credits were recorded on a 3½-by-5½-inch card divided into separate earning and spending sections. Each section had 200 credits divided into twenty columns of ten credits each. Both earnings and expenditures were recorded by means of a punch whose extremely complex pattern reduced the probability of cheating since it could not be easily duplicated.

The number of credits dispensed for each job varied from one to four depending upon the amount of effort required to complete each job. The number of credits required to purchase the system's special items and privileges also varied depending upon their costs to the unit.

Each patient carried not only his own earning and spending card, but also the job cards corresponding to those jobs that he had been assigned. The bottom section of each job card had twelve spaces corresponding to Monday through Saturday for a two-week period. The cards were arranged in chronological order and were secured by a small, screw-type binding post placed through holes in the upper right hand corner of each card. Multicolored fabric pouches were given to each patient for storage of the cards. When a job was appropriately completed, the supervising staff member punched both the space on the job card that corresponded to the day on which the job was successfully completed and the appropriate number of credits on the earning and spending card.

Data Collection

It was thought that the use of the cards would simplify data collection procedures since the act of supervision was to have terminated in both reinforcement and data recording. However, patients began to lose their card packets at the collective rate of approximately one packet per day in spite of the fact that they were charged twenty-five credits to make up a new packet. Unfortunately, a lost packet resulted in lost data. In addition, not only did the punching process leave small bits of litter scattered about the unit's floor, but the design of the earning and spending card did not allow for quick and accurate determination of the amount of credits that were available for spending.

Hence, it was decided to switch back to tokens and maintain the job board as the system's major organizational and scheduling device. A new data system was then devised which consisted of four 8½-by-14-inch sheets on which each job is chronologically listed in the rows, and each day of a two-week period in the columns. In addition, there is a space next to each job in which the name of the patient to whom it has been assigned can be written. Thus, the data sheets in large part duplicate the job board.

After supervision of a routine has been completed, the staff member completes the data sheet using the following scale:

0: not available to prompt;
1: did not show up;
2: showed up, attempted no work, or attempted some work, but did not redo;
3: attempted to work and redo the job, but did not do the job correctly or did not complete the redo in time;
4: showed up, did the job correctly after having to redo the job; and
5: did the job correctly without having to redo.

Figure VI-1 presents the first of the four data sheets.

The system is assessed and jobs reassigned every two weeks. The principal criterion for reassignment is a completion rate of

Do not dispense credit for 0, 1, 2, 3

0: Not available to prompt
1: Did not show up
2: Showed up, attempted no work, or attempted some work, but did not redo
3: Attempted to work and redo the job, but did not do the job correctly or did not complete the redo in time

Dispense credit for .4 and 5

4: Showed up did the job correctly after having to redo the job
5: Did the job correctly without having to redo

Put the appropriate performance level in the box:

— Days —

Patient	Job	Credit	T	W	Th	F	S	Free	M	T	W	Th	F	S	Free	M	
	Up and clothes on																NOC
	Up and clothes on																
	Up and clothes on																
	Up and clothes on																
	Up and clothes on																
	Up and clothes on																
	Up and clothes on																
	Up and clothes on																
	Up and clothes on																
	Up and clothes on																
	Up and clothes on																
	Up and clothes on																

Figure VI-1. (continued on next page)

less than 80 percent. Such a completion rate results in reassignment to a less difficult task which is accomplished by reshuffling patient name cards on the job board and by writing on the data sheet the name of the new patient to whom the job has been assigned.

Patient	Job	Credit	T	W	Th	F	S	Free	M	T	W	Th	F	S	Free	M
	Groom															
	Groom															
	Groom															
	Groom															
	Groom															
	Groom															
	Groom															
	Groom															
	Groom															
	Groom															
	Groom															
	Groom															
	Get trash can & fix 2 dishwaters															
	Get food cart															
	Serve plates															
	Set table w/ utensils and milk															
	Ready cart to return															
	Return cart															
	Clean tables & empty trash															
* *	* * * *	*	*	*	*	*	*	*	*	*	*	*	*	*	*
	Wash & dry chairs															
	Put up chairs															
	Sweep & mop dining room															
	Put down dining room chairs															

Figure VI-1.   The first of four data collection sheets.

Staff Behavior

A number of training sessions were held to acquaint the staff with the new system, explain the job board, and specify the behaviors they were to emit in order to effectively implement the system. Basically, staff members assume responsibility for supervising only one routine at a time. They gather all of the appropriate materials at the site before the routine begins, and then they instruct each patient involved in the routine that it is time to do his job. Those patients who appear at the job site are given the materials; after indicating that the job is completed, the job performance is compared to the listed criteria. The patient is given one opportunity to correct a deficient performance, after which the job is rechecked. Token reinforcement and a minimum of thirty seconds of social reinforcement is dispensed if the job performance meets the criteria. Social reinforcement is defined as providing eye contact, speaking in a pleasant tone of voice, and maintaining some type of physical contact such as a touch on the shoulder.

When the system was first implemented, there was some difficulty in maintaining appropriate staff behavior. The unit's charge nurse was absent at that time because of illness, and the day shift (7:45 A.M. to 5:15 P.M.) was primarily staffed by two trainees who had been placed on the CRU from other units in the hospital to receive three months of intensive training. Unfortunately, these two trainees had to discharge regular CRU duties which they were not well equipped to handle.

When the charge nurse returned to the unit, she was briefed about the system and began to emit the appropriate behavior. Other staff members soon followed suit. An earlier study had indicated the effects of the charge nurse's modeling appropriate behavior as compared to giving instructions and removing competing activities (Wallace, et al., 1973). In that study, nursing staff members interacted with patients only when the behavior was modeled by either the charge nurse or by the unit's professional staff. Neither instructions nor the removal of competing activities had any effect on their rate of interaction.

INTERFACE WITH OTHER SYSTEMS

The token economy interfaces with the other systems principally through the use of the token as a generalized reinforcer. Thus, the individualized system may use tokens to consequate a behavior which is not normally part of the token economy. For example, tokens may be used to reward on-task remarks during assertion training, appropriate approaches during social interaction, etc. These behaviors are defined, recorded, and consequated, however, as part of the individualized system.

The use of tokens in the individualized system also allows token earnings to be equated across patients with differential ability to successfully complete the tasks of the economy. A patient who is only able to groom may be rewarded with tokens for an individually targeted behavior such as answering a simple question. This gives him an opportunity to earn as many tokens as the patient who is able to successfully complete any and all tasks of the economy.

SUMMARY

With the introduction of the job board the token economy was considerably simplified and standardized. Data is now completed at approximately a 95-percent rate and comments from the nursing staff indicate that the board is quite helpful, particularly if anyone occasionally has to work a different shift. Reassignment of jobs is quite easy, and the economy seems to function smoothly and efficiently.

REFERENCES

Wallace, C. J.; Davis, J. R.; Liberman, R. P., and Baker, V.: Modeling and staff behavior. *J Consult Clin Psychol, 41*:422, 1973.

MOVEMENT AND GOAL DIRECTION WITHIN TOKEN ECONOMIES

JOHN M. ATTHOWE, JR., PH.D.

In 1962, TOGETHER with Len Krasner, the author began a behavior modification unit at the V.A. Hospital in Palo Alto (Atthowe and Krasner, 1968). Due to the newness and thus controversial nature of the project, we were assigned an eighty-six-bed chronic back ward consisting largely of chronic regressed schizophrenics and the brain damaged. The average length of hospitalization was twenty-two years and the median age was fifty-seven years. Most of the patients were seen as requiring continual supervision (i.e. an aide accompanied them on all off-ward activities).

As in most large hospitals, everyone had given up on these patients. The only form of treatment was substantial maintenance doses of medication. At first a number of the new behavior therapy techniques were tried with a limited number of patients. It was found that relaxation training, systematic desensitization, assertive training, and aversive conditioning generally had a limited effect and were quite time-consuming with this population. The use of contingent reinforcement procedures, especially positive reinforcement, showed some gains for very specific types of target behaviors but were not readily maintained nor generalized. It was almost impossible first to find, and secondly to provide, reinforcers that remained potent or that could be administered either immediately or routinely. Thus, it was decided to utilize token reinforcements and develop a token economy for the entire unit.

133

DEVELOPING A TOKEN PROGRAM

In developing the ward token economy, it was necessary to first secure the acceptance of the already existing ward staff. This was not easy and necessitated a one-year training period which served as a convenient operant baseline. During this training period there were frequent staff meetings in which the basic tenets of the future program were explained and the more detailed ideas worked out; meanwhile, everyone became involved in observing and recording behavioral episodes. At this stage in the implementation of the program it became apparent that the success of a token economy or any total hospital program is laregly dependent upon the cooperation of the entire ward staff and, in particular, those members of the nursing staff who would carry out the program (i.e. the psychiatric aides). In addition, each mental health discipline had its own implicit as well as explicit system of contingencies or social system. Thus, in order to bring about the acceptance of the program, it was necessary to shape or "sell" each of the different services and disciplines from nursing and psychiatry to dietetics and recreation.

In the process of recording baseline data it was found that what was done on the ward could easily be undone off the ward by others who failed to carry out the same program with the same degree of interest and enthusiasm. If an effective token program was to be developed and maintained, it was also essential to include all the relevant hospital social systems in the program. The persons who controlled the contingencies and dispensed the reinforcements for the patient population were many and varied both on and off the ward. Thus, the primary target of the ward program during the long baseline phase turned out to be those who dispensed the reinforcement—the hospital staff.

The extended baseline period also provided clues regarding the impact of certain environmental events. For example, the Christmas season markedly disrupted the performance of many patients. The number of patients not getting up in the morning on time markedly increased as did withdrawal and irritability. Furthermore, it became apparent that patients who were becoming high or depressed could be spotted before this latter behavior became obvious by observing an increase in the number of infractions in their base rates. When the systematic contingencies (tokens) were introduced, these variations were not as great nor as readily spotted; however, during the first Christmas period under the token program, early morning infractions, which had been steadily decreasing, rose markedly from eighteen to thirty-nine.

THE ART OF SHAPING

Operating a token economy is more than following a set of rules or procedures. The effective administration of reinforcers necessitated knowing the social (contingency) systems operating in general and at any given time. The relationships of staff to patients, of patients to patients, and of administrative personnel to both staff and patients were different and unique, giving different weight to each reinforcing occasion, so that at different times identical reinforcers might have different results. We found that explicit contingencies must be maintained and that unique or excessive punishment for not carrying out an activity is best avoided. If patients began to give up on the system and earn fewer and fewer tokens, their overall performance deteriorated. If records are kept of the patient's daily or weekly performance, drops in effectiveness can be quickly caught and individualized programs initiated. It is at this point that individualized shaping can become the major therapeutic procedure.

Imposing an invariable set of contingencies (rules and regulations) upon a program automatically dooms it. Such a program will soon reach a stabilized way of operating, and eventually the reinforcers and the contingent behaviors will lose their potency. This is why a token economy must be a continually changing program in which different opportunities and reinforcers are alway being programmed. The "art" of shaping (Sidman, 1962) is the most important therapeutic tool within the token program.

Excesses should be avoided in the operation of a token economy. If patients are given too many fines or pile up a sizeable debt of tokens, they soon drop out of the program.

If some patients earn and keep a large number of tokens on hand or in a bank, they become independent of the therapeutic milieu. The purpose of a token program is not patient management but the development of therapeutic movement. The goal of any therapeutic program is improvement in one's functioning. In a token economy this entails shaping, the delicate art of balancing rewards and non-rewards, of delaying the administration of reinforcement as the patient improves, of reducing or enlarging the amount and the scope of the reinforcement, etc. Shaping entails continual movement toward some goal. In most hospital token economies this short-term goal is increased motivation or activity.

THE GOALS OF SHAPING

The most frequently put forth and most readily attainable short-term goal of shaping within a token economy is an increase in activity or motivation. In particular settings, this goal may shift to the elimination of undesirable behaviors and the substitution of more desirable responses. Another short-term goal of shaping is more directly related to staff satisfaction and, as such, raises potential ethical issues. This is the goal of management, whether it be better classroom or ward control. A point can be made that better management creates the possibility of more effective therapeutic intervention; and in this sense, a more efficiently operating and well-managed token program has a greater chance of producing therapeutic change. But better management in and of itself should not be a goal of shaping. The courts hold that a goal of management, *per se,* for non-voluntary, institutionalized individuals conflicts with the patient's right to treatment (Mental Health Law Project, 1973).

A longer-term goal of the shaping process with institutionalized individuals is getting the person out of the institution. One of the goals of treatment is to return the deviant child to his regular classroom, the felon and the mental patient back to society, and the retardate to a more productive and satisfying life outside the confines of an institution. The attainment of this goal has not met with overwhelming success; however, the few comparative studies to date indicate that token economies are more likely to bring this about than other therapeutic programs (Hall and Baker, 1973; Heap, et al., 1970; Kazdin and Bootzin, 1972; O'Leary and Drabman, 1971).

The goals of shaping will vary with the population considered and the nature of the problem. Ultimately, however, the goal all programs seek is to produce better functioning individuals and to maintain and perpetuate this improvement. There seems to be little doubt that more often than not better functioning can be produced. Bringing about effective or "normal" functioning is harder, but attainable. The persistence or maintenance of these changes, however, has been hard to demonstrate (Atthowe, 1973; Kazdin and Bootzin, 1972). It is now time to pay closer attention to the long-term goals of shaping within token economies, that is, the persistence of effective functioning.

MOVING MENTAL PATIENTS INTO THE COMMUNITY

The most difficult and costly diagnosis to treat in the mental health field is the chronic mental patient whether this patient is psychotic or definitely brain damaged. More time and effort is spent on a few hard-core long-term patients than with any other patient group (Decker and Stubblebine, 1972; Smith, et al., 1974). Furthermore, the longer one is hospitalized, the less likely he will ever leave the confines of that institution. Within five years, the likelihood of returning to the community is less than one in twenty (Fairweather, et al., 1960).

In spite of such pessimistic findings, we began to encounter more and more success in changing the behavior of chronic schizophrenics within the institution; therefore, we started to look at longer-term goals. It was found that the majority of patients could eventually move into more active and therapeutically advanced programs and twice as many patients were being discharged. Yet, we had not really developed a program designed to discharge patients. The recidivism rate of our program was also fairly high (approximately 50%), although it was below the base rate (around 60-70%) for similar V.A. hospitals.

It became obvious that if our goal was to discharge patients and keep them out of the hospital, such a goal should be explicitly involved in the treatment plans. However, we wanted not only to maintain people within the community but also to train them to be independent and self-sufficient, to be productive members of their community.

Our long-term goals became the discharge of patients, their maintenance outside of the institution and their development of a productive and self-sufficient community existence. Three factors gave us cues in developing our plans. One factor was the powerful reinforcing condition of a step system in our original token program. A second factor was that those patients who reached or were in the process of reaching the top step (the ward's elite group) were invariably working in meaningful jobs which were similar in nature if not in pressure to jobs outside the hospital. The third factor was the existence of a program mainly designed to reduce recidivism. This program not only incorporated a group step system within the treatment milieu but also created a maintaining milieu outside the institution (Fairweather, et al., 1969). These investigators created both a sheltered work program (e.g. a housecleaning business) and a sheltered living arrangement (a motel) within the community. One of the investigators directed the work program out of the motel.

MOVEMENT BY STEPS

As we noted previously, a successful program must involve movement toward some end, and the best means of accomplishing such movement is the shaping process in which prompting, reinforcement, fading and thinning are interwoven into a goal-directed program. Within a token economy, shaping large groups is greatly facilitated by a step or levels system.

Not all patients respond to changes in their therapeutic milieu in the same way or at the same rate. Consequently, it seems a bit dehumanizing and is very inefficient to reward all patients for shaving or dressing appropriately or to send all patients to "art therapy." Many patients would move too fast through the system and stabilize their performance or learn to "beat the system." Other patients would move too slowly, become frustrated (as would the staff) and eventually not respond to the system. Therefore, in shaping large groups of people, a step or levels system is an important adjunct so that enthusiasm and interest can be maintained from the initiation of the program to its culmination. A step system makes it possible for each patient to advance at his own pace.

In observing the performance of the original group of chronic patients (Atthowe and Krasner, 1968) during the baseline period, three general performance classes emerged. The largest group, approximately 60 percent, required continual attention and supervision. They could not go off the ward alone without wandering and getting lost. Almost all of these men had to be cajoled into taking care of themselves and dressing properly. They were inactive, completely unmotivated with few, if any, wants, and unresponsive to the social milieu of which they were a part. A second group of patients (about 25%) were more responsive and motivated. They had ground privileges and could go off the ward unescorted. They tended to attend the activities provided for them during the day and were socially responsive to the staff and to a few of their peers. The third group (approximately 15%) required only minimal supervision and had learned how to adapt to the hospital environment. They were fairly self-sufficient within the protective environment of the hospital. They were socially responsive to the staff and to other patients, and usually had acquired certain patterns of behavior that paid off within the hospital milieu. Some of these patients enjoyed going on passes, but they had an excessive fear of ever leaving the protection of the hospital. The outside world is and was aversive to them, and the staff seldom gave them any guidance or training that would counteract these fears. This fear became one of the major obstacles in the movement of patients back to the community.

At first, everyone was rewarded when he carried out the basic contingency program (see Appendix A). It soon became apparent, however, that patients at the lowest performance level (Level III) found it hard to acquire tokens; consequently, they did very little. Thus, staff members were asked to spend more time with this group and to reinforce them immediately whenever their behavior approximated desirable performance. On the other hand, Level II patients had no trouble acquiring tokens if they were motivated to do so. Their desires and wants were much greater, and they could bridge a delay in the acquisition of tokens or their backup reinforcers. Therefore, it was of little or no consequence to this group to receive a token for shaving. It was more rewarding to receive a batch of tokens on a "token payday" once a week than to be under the close supervision of staff members who were prompting, instructing, and reinforcing the carrying out of the activities of daily living. Level I patients could probably function in a boarding home outside the confines of the institution if they were so trained. They were much more socially responsible and able to participate in work assignments. If they were put in with Level III patients, Level I patients would find the situation very degrading and either work themselves out of their predicament rapidly or drop out of the program. Consequently, many patients were begun at Level II.

Initially, differences in performance were tied to the magnitude of the backup reinforcers. The concept of a balance between the number of tokens earned and the number spent is one of the more important rules of thumb in developing a token economy. If many tokens are earned and not spent, therapeutic movement (shaping) is diminished. If only a few tokens are earned and many more are needed to satisfy an individual's wants, positive movement is stopped and tangential goals become important. Thus, Level III patients' low performances were linked to their wants which were more basic and physiological in nature. For example, two of the more important reinforcers for Level III patients were a pack of cigarettes and staying on the ward (i.e. sitting in overstuffed chairs); both activities were worth only two tokens. Appendix B presents the token costs of the backup reinforcers. It can be seen that as the ability to earn tokens increased, the cost of things that would interest Level II patients was also increased. By the time patients were stimulated to take passes and become more independent, prices of backup reinforcers reflected their increased earning power. It also can be seen that patients were encouraged to seek out new reinforcing activities by having free time to watch television, play table tennis or pool, stay on the ward, etc. To be able to get something at a bargain is especially motivating, even for chronic patients. In order to shape persons in the direction of leaving the hospital on a pass, money was tied to passes. If a patient wished to receive two dollars without going on a pass, it would cost him twenty tokens; however, he could also receive two dollars for twelve tokens if a day pass of less than four hours was taken.

Level I patients were a special and select group. They were both in and out of the token program. They had to earn their way into the group and thus out of the token program. The main requirement was the accumulation of 120 tokens which meant at least three weeks of full-time work and the denial of some immediate gratifications. Upon becoming a member of this elite group, patients were given a special token or card (a "carte blanche") which entitled the bearer to all of the backup reinforcers available to ward members without the hassle of performing daily for staff members, attending a token payday, or planning how to spend their limited resources for the next week. In addition, Level I patients were given extra privileges (see Table VII-I). However, Level I patients were also expected to work at least twenty-five hours per week in a meaningful job, be a "buddy" to another patient on the ward, not violate general ward or hospital rules, and submit a plan for leaving the hospital. Usually all of these patients worked in the rehabilitation program of the on-the-grounds Veterans Workshop which contracted work such as restoration of old telephones, etc.

The token economy program was designed to move the patient from Level III to Level I by making each succeeding step much more attractive. However, a number of patients became very ambivalent about moving to the next higher level, especially if the next level required a lessening of institutionalized dependency and a focus upon leaving the hospital. Consequently, movement into Level I often was not automatic and required considerable prompting to overcome the fear associated with leaving the hospital.

Other programs employing levels systems (Fairweather, 1964;

TABLE VII-I

Group A patients' white card will gain all the privileges given to those on the token system plus these extra privileges: (a) leaving for and getting into the dining hall first at every meal, (b) sitting together in the dining hall at a special table, (c) sleeping in a special area where the lights do not go on until 6:30 A.M., (d) receiving extra passes every day, except Monday and Wednesday, from 4 P.M. to 5 P.M., (e) receiving automatic passes on the weekend from 4 P.M. on Friday to 11 P.M. Sunday (everyone must sign up on the pass list by Tuesday in order to get day and weekend passes and/or medication), (f) receiving 50 cents per hour for work at the Veteran's Work Shop, (g) anyone in Group A for 30 days may ask for a discharge or LOA (leave of absence) at any time, and (h) bank their money in town.

Kelley and Henderson, 1971; Schaefer and Martin, 1969) have also stressed the acquisition of behaviors that are more like those needed outside the hospital plus the fading or thinning out of the tokens or their equivalent. Fairweather and his colleagues (1964) in a contingent, nontoken program introduced the notion of group movement in an effort to stimulate social responsiveness and social pressure among their patients. Four levels were predicated, and movement depended upon the performance of the entire group. If one patient within the group failed to respond, the entire group suffered; thus, group members tended to police their own groups. For many individuals group pressure is a greater incentive than individualized pressure. This is especially true for patients akin to our Levels I and II. However, self-pacing is minimized in a group contingency program and Level III patients do not function well in such a program. A Level II, paranoid patient who was in both the token program described above (Atthowe and Krasner, 1968) and in the Fairweather group program (Fairweather, 1964) categorized both programs as follows: "I like the token program because it is capitalistic. You get what you do. The group program is communistic, you only get what the group gets."

Some of the problems that frequently arise in shaping and in moving patients from one level or step to another are due to the lack of specificity of the steps and the lack of communication of this specificity. If one initially makes an analysis of the programs' goals he can then develop subgoals or steps that are readily attainable. Frequent, relevant, and manageable subgoals and steps are necessary for patient movement. If an individual patient stops moving, an individually tailored program may be superimposed upon the overall program. One of the better ways to define the subgoals of a program is to think in terms of the behaviors that a person should be performing at each step or subgoal enroute to the terminal goal (Houts and Scott, 1972). Houts and Scott provide these considerations: (1) If possible involve the patient, (2) set goals that are achievable (i.e. manageable steps), (3) specify the goal by describing what the patient will be doing or how he will be acting when the goal is achieved, (4) set a date when the goal should be reached, and (5) describe the treatment plan clearly and specifically in working toward the goal.

DEVELOPING MANAGEABLE STEPS

In a recent review of mental hospital programs, Anthony, et al. (1972), concluded that, "Traditional methods of treating hospitalized psychiatric patients, including individual therapy, group therapy, work therapy and drug therapy, do not effect differentially the discharged patients' community functioning as measured by recidivism and post-hospital employment" (p. 454). Token programs are a bit more effective than these therapies, but the problem remains. How do we move patients out of the hospital, and how can we keep them from returning?

As we indicated earlier, Fairweather and his colleagues (Fairweather, et al., 1969) kept patients out in the community and working by actually taking treatment into the community. By setting up a self-contained community project (a halfway house and work program), they were able to increase the amount of time spent in the community from 24 percent (control group) to 65 percent, and the rate of employment from 3 to 50 percent. However, the step from a hospital ward to independent living is too big a step for many patients, especially chronic patients, without specialized training and guidance at successive stages in this process. Fairweather and his colleagues' results did indicate that if one desired a certain terminal behavior to be performed, then one must create the occasion for that behavior to be performed and reinforce it.

Expanding on the ideas of Fairweather (Fairweather, et al., 1969) and the notion of shaping, a series of steps were developed that were readily attainable, graduated, specific, and meaningful (i.e. chained or tied to the ultimate goal of independent and self-sufficient living). The program was called "Operation Reentry" (Atthowe, 1973; Atthowe and McDonough, 1969).

As patients progressed through the token program to the status of Group I patients, they not only earned their way out of the token system, but also went to work in a sheltered workshop on the hospital grounds. The workshop, a nonprofit corporation (see McDonough, 1969), provided patients with a number of meaningful jobs which were designed to approximate the performance level of a patient at any given time. A few patients merely bundled newspapers, others nailed crates or polished telephones and cleaned telephone cords or painted. In addition, a number of off-the-grounds work programs were instituted, such as house renovation, gardening, and gas station operation. These latter kinds of jobs provided training in the activities patients would be expected to be performing when discharged. We have found that those patients who worked were less likely to return to the hospital. At first, patients were paid quite nominal or therapeutic wages. As patients progressed within the program, their wages increased. In some of the work programs in 1971, patients were earning more than four dollars per hour. Money, status, comradeship, social reinforcement, and self-reinforcement (greater environmental mastery and self-reliance) increased at each successive step.

In other words, as a patient advanced through the program token reinforcements were increased, thinned out, and eventually superceded by natural reinforcers. The natural reinforcers in turn increased in value as the patient assumed more responsibility. At the same time the patient's living arrangements were noticeably improved. At first patients lived in large dormitories. As they earned more tokens they could buy their way into more private quarters and eventually into Group I. Group I, the elite group, was quartered in a separate area of the ward opened only to those patients. They had their own day room and television and arranged their living and sleeping areas according to their own desires. Recidivism was found to decrease if Group I patients were moved to a special self-help ward before discharge rather than being discharged directly. Living on the self-help ward was more like living in a halfway house than a regular ward. Patients assumed more responsibility for their own lives. They worked in the sheltered workshop programs both on the grounds and off. They took their own medication (occasionally the taking of medication was checked by chemical tests). No staff people were allowed on the ward except for one therapist who ran group therapy sessions. Therapy consisted of a review of progress, information, job and post-hospital orientation, and everyday problems encountered at work and in getting along with others.

It was found in a survey of discharged patients at this and other V.A. hospitals that loneliness was the major factor in bringing people back to the hospital. As the ex-patient became more and more lonely, he isolated himself, drank more, and stopped taking medication. Movement out of the hospital in groups seems to be one answer to this problem. Consequently, the patients were assigned to groups of four to six on the self-help ward. These groups became the basis for therapy and movement into the community. It was suggested, but never implemented, that a small house be set up on the grounds which the small groups would first move into and encounter the problems of everyday living, before moving off the grounds. Instead, as a first step off the ward, a number of three-bedroom houses near the hospital were rented and patients moved into the community in groups of five. Later, apartments were rented in the same housing complex, and groups of two were assigned to each apartment.

Thus, a graduated series of steps was developed from traditional ward activities to special privileges and greater responsibility within the ward, to a self-help and more independent ward. The step off the grounds was facilitated by the creation of group cohesion and group pressure. Small groups of patients were formed and lived together, first on a self-help ward (quarterway house), and then in a rented home in the outside community (three-quarterway house). The use of a halfway house, a small house on the grounds, was conceptualized but never materialized; however, in the ideal step-system it would be a necessary phase. At each step the behaviors necessary for patients to maintain themselves at that step and the next succeeding steps were taught. In order to overcome some of the resistance to living in the community, ex-patients who were living outside the hospital worked side by side with patients in workshop jobs. In this sense, the ex-patient served as a positive model. At other times a few of these ex-patients volunteered to act as group leaders or co-therapists in the therapy groups. We found the peer therapist to be more effective in overcoming the fear of leaving the hospital than a staff member whose job was seen as getting patients out of the hospital. The use of peers as therapists not only helped to get patients oriented to getting out, but also helped the ex-patient to stay out.

Each step in the program is viewed as a step enroute to the ultimate goal of self-sufficient and effective functioning. Progress can be measured in terms of nearness to the ultimate goal, time in the community, time working, and the quality of work performed. The explicit designation of what behaviors define each step or subgoal makes it possible to scale the degree of attainment of the next step and whether or not progress is being made. The recidivism rate over one year was less than 12 percent (Atthowe, 1973) as compared with a much higher rate (60 to 70%) for other V.A. hospital patients. In addition, all of these ex-patients worked forty hours per week. It seems that as long as the ex-patient can be desensitized to moving into the community through experience and training and observing others who have succeeded, as long as they advance in small manageable steps, and as long as they live and work together in small groups in a supportive community, the likelihood of moving out of the institution and staying out is greatly increased. As the patient gains confidence and new skills he can venture more and more on his own with the knowledge that peers are not too far away. All hospital programs, including token economies, are both rehabilitation and habilitation programs in which the shaping of the newly-asked-for behaviors and mastery goes hand in hand with a lessening of hospital control and of constructed contingencies.

The broader the range of contingencies within the program and the greater the frequency of natural reinforcers, the greater the chances for persistence. If we make persistence a goal *per se,* then we need to create the environment we desire and the maintaining milieu, and to reinforce their perpetuation. Shaping and fading are our two most important tools. We cannot lessen our support too soon nor maintain it too long.

Appendix A
WAYS OF EARNING TOKENS

I. On Ward (Daily)
- A. Getting up on time, making bed, and being downstairs by 7:15 A.M. (given at door when leaving for breakfast) — 1 token
- B. *Shaving* and combing hair (given at ward canteen) — 1 token
- C. Clothes clean and dressed neatly (given at ward canteen) — 1 token
- D. Bed and bed area neat and clean (given at noon medication) — 1 token
- E. Pouring water during medications — 1 token each time
- F. *Helping* on ward, such as running errands — 1 token/errand
- G. Going to scheduled *appointments* off the ward and bringing back an initialed appointment card to secretary's office — 2 tokens
- H. Housekeeping and cleaning on the ward at any time — 2 tokens/hour
- I. If two or more patients play cards, checkers, pool or table tennis together on the ward, for at least half an hour during the following hours: 11 A.M. to 12:30 P.M. and 1:30 to 10 P.M. — 2 tokens/hour
- J. *Pension* for being over seventy years old (given at ward canteen) — 3 tokens

II. On Ward (Weekly)
- A. Taking a *shower* between 3:30 and 5 P.M. on Monday, Wednesday, and Friday (given when you receive your new clothes in clothing room) — 1 token each time
- B. Attending *ward meeting* when scheduled — 1 token
- C. Attending your scheduled *group meeting* — 2 tokens
- D. Running movie *projector* — 3 tokens each time
- E. Being ward representative to Patient's Congress (given Tuesday at 9 A.M.) — 3 tokens/week
- F. Being *Acorn* reporter for ward (given Tuesday at 9 A.M.) — 3 tokens/week
- G. In charge of making coffee during group meeting or popcorn in evening — 3 tokens each time
- H. Attending *treatment* or therapy session — 4 tokens

III. Off-ward Activities
- A. *Attending group activities* (art, swimming, RT in gym, ET, golf, OT, CT, RT on Tuesday and Thursday evening and weekend movies) — 1 token/hour
- B. Attending and participating in *group activities* — 2 tokens/hour
- C. Participating in *individual assignments* such as MAT activities, library, art sketch trip (given Tuesday at 9 A.M.) — 2 tokens/hour

148

D. Attending *I.T. Assignments*: The first ten hours per week will be worth two tokens per hour; each hour after that will be worth three tokens per hour if rating is fair or better (given Tuesday at 9 A.M.)

IV. Special Bonuses

A.	If weekly I.T. rating is *Good* (given Tuesday at 9 A.M.)	3 tokens
B.	If weekly I.T. rating is *Very Good* (given Tuesday at 9 A.M.)	7 tokens
C.	*Writing* an article for the *Acorn*	9 tokens
D.	*Representing* the ward in some activity off the ward	6 tokens
E.	Any reasonable *suggestion* for new additions to the token program	15 tokens
F.	Anyone with a pass card who takes a patient without a pass card off the grounds on an accompanied pass	10 tokens

Appendix B

COST OF THINGS

I. In Ward Canteen

1 pack of cigarettes	2 tokens
1 cigar	1 token
1 pack of tobacco	1 token
10 cents worth of canteen coupons	
Any other item in canteen	1 token

II. On Ward (Daily Activities)

A. To *stay on ward* from 9 to 11 A.M. and 2 to 3 P.M. (Sunday is free) — 2 tokens/hour

B. To watch television from 7 A.M. to 10 P.M. — 1 token/hour

C. To *leave the ward in the evenings,* or obtain other evening privileges — 3 tokens

D. To *go early to meals* with Group A, ten minutes before the ward goes — 2 tokens

E. To see ward physician, nurse, social worker or psychologist; patients must first get an appointment card from the ward secretary which costs

F. To play pool or table tennis (Sunday is free) — 1 token/hour

G. To bring cartons of milk or other *food items on ward* (food not allowed upstairs) — 1 token/item

H. To get up and *shave or go downstairs before 6 A.M.* — 1 token

III. On Ward (Weekly Activities)

A. To see *evening movies* on ward — 1 token

B. To *sleep till 7 on Sunday morning* — 1 token in advance

C. To *sleep in certain bed areas:*

In Group A alcove (lights on at 6:30 A.M.)	12 tokens/week
Six-bed alcove in south wing (lights on at 6:20)	9 tokens/week
Two-bed alcove in hall (lights on at 6:20)	9 tokens/week
Large south wing (lights on at 6:10)	6 tokens/week
Large north wing (lights on at 6)	3 tokens/week

IV. Money and Passes (Paid for Every Tuesday)

A. *Weekly cash* for those not going on a pass (maximum limit $10) Each 10 cents equals — 1 token

B. Special cash will be given for a specific purpose on the following basis:

1. Up to $5	6 tokens
2. Up to $10	10 tokens
3. Up to $20	20 tokens
4. Over $20	30 tokens

C. *Passes* (passes and cash go together)

1. A day pass of less than *four hours* and up to a maximum of $2 — 12 tokens

2. An *accompanied* day pass and up to a
   maximum of $5   15 tokens
3. A *day pass* and up to a maximum of $5   25 tokens
4. An *overnight pass* and up to a maximum of
   $10   35 tokens
5. An *accompanied weekend pass* and up to a
   maximum of $5   30 tokens
6. *Weekend pass* (2 nights out) and up to a
   maximum of $20   50 tokens
7. For an *extended pass,* up to five nights, each
   additional night beyond two nights will be   25 tokens
8. A *leave of absence* from seven to fourteen
   days   125 tokens
9. A *leave of absence* from fifteen to thirty days 175 tokens
10. A ninety-day *trial visit* requires that a person
    be in Group A for thirty days   175 tokens

D. Special Passes
   1. Recreational outings   10 tokens
   2. Red Cross rides   6 tokens
   3. Special off-station activities   Dependent on activity

REFERENCES

Anthony, W. A.; Buell, G. J.; Sharratt, S., and Althoff, M. E.: Efficacy of psychiatric rehabilitation. *Psychol Bull*, 78:447, 1972.

Atthowe, J. M., Jr.: Behavior innovation and persistence. *Am Psychol*, 28:34, 1973.

Atthowe, J. M., Jr., and Krasner, L.: A preliminary report on the application of contingent reinforcement procedures (token economy) on a "chronic" psychiatric ward. *J Abnorm Psychol*, 73:37, 1968.

Atthowe, J. M., Jr., and McDonough, J. M.: *Operations Re-entry* (film of V.A. Hospital, Palo Alto, Calif.; released by Indiana University). Washington, D.C., U.S. Department of Health, Education and Welfare, Social and Rehabilitation Services, 1969.

Decker, J. B., and Stubblebine, J. M.: Crisis intervention and prevention of psychiatric disability. *Am J Psychiatry*, 129:725, 1972.

Fairweather, G. W. (Ed.): *Social Psychology in Treating Mental Illness: An Experimental Approach*. New York, Wiley, 1964.

Fairweather, G. W.; Sanders, D. H.; Crissler, D. L., and Maynard, A.: *Community Life for the Mentally Ill*. Chicago, Aldine, 1969.

Fairweather, G. W.; Simon, R.; Bebhard, M. E.; Weingarten, E.; Holland, J. L.; Sanders, R.; Stone, G. B., and Reahl ,J. E.: Relative effectiveness of psychotherapeutic programs: A multicriteria comparison of four programs for three different patient groups. *Psychol Monogr*, 74 (5, whole No. 492): 1960, 1-26.

Hall, J., and Baker, R.: Token economy systems: Breakdown and control. *Behav Res Ther*, 11:253, 1973.

Heap, R. F.; Boblitt, W. E.; Moore, C. H., and Hord, J. E.: Behavior-milieu therapy with chronic neuropsychiatric patients. *J Abnorm Psychol*, 76:349, 1970.

Houts, P. S., and Scott, R. A.: *Goal Planning in Mental Health Rehabilitation*. Hershey, The Milton S. Hershey Medical Center, 1972.

Kazdin, A. E., and Bootzin, R. R.: The token economy: An evaluation review. *J Appl Behav Anal*, 5:543, 1972.

Kelley, K. M., and Henderson, J. D.: A community-based operant learning environment II: Systems and procedures. In Rubin, R. D.; Fensterheim, H.; Lazarus, A. A., and Franks, C. M. (Eds.): *Advances in Behavior Therapy*. New York, Acad Pr, 1971.

McDonough, J. M.: The Veterans Administration and Community Mental Health: New approaches in psychiatric rehabilitation. *Community Ment Health J*, 5:275, 1969.

Mental Health Law Project: *Basic Rights of the Mentally Handicapped.* Washington, D.C., Mental Health Law Project, 1973.

O'Leary, K. D., and Drabman, R.: Token reinforcement programs in the classroom: A review. *Psychol Bull, 75*:379, 1971.

Schaefer, H. H., and Martin, P. L.: *Behavioral Therapy.* New York, McGraw, 1969.

Sidman, M.: Operant techniques .In Bachrach, A. J.: *Experimental Foundations of Clinical Psychology.* New York, Basic, 1962, pp. 170-210.

Smith, W. G.; Kaplan, J., and Siker, D.: Community Mental Health and the seriously disturbed patient. *Arch Gen Psychiatry, 30*:693, 1974.

THE PUNCH CARD TOKEN
ECONOMY PROGRAM*

JOHN PAUL FOREYT, PH.D.

WHILE THERE IS almost unanimous agreement that token economies modify the behavior of patients in mental institutions, evaluations of these programs generally show that 10 to 20 percent of patients in these programs do not respond to the reinforcement procedures. Many of these failures are due to either an inadequately trained staff or an economy not functioning as tightly as possible.

Ideally, a new program director would like to be able to select his aides and other staff members and adequately train them before the program begins. In reality, however, the new program director will probably be given a hospital back ward with the staff members already there (in fact, many will have been on that ward before the program director was born), and he will be told to set up his token economy.

There are several major problems he must resolve immediately. The most important one involves the question of *authority*. To run an effective program, the director must be able to act on the numerous day-to-day problems that occur on his ward. Although he is probably a psychologist, the staff members on his ward are psychiatric aides, supervised by a nurse, responsible to the director of nursing. If the director of nursing has the

* The token economy program at Florida State Hospital, Chattahoochee, Florida, is supported by a Department of Health, Education, and Welfare Public Health Service Hospital Improvement Program Grant (04-R-000013-01-1).

power to arbitrarily transfer trained staff members out of the program, replacing them with untrained aides, or insist that her aides wear white uniforms rather than street clothes, etc., the program director will find himself spending all his time fighting the director of nursing rather than training his staff to work with patients. If the clinical director of the hospital refuses to allow patients grounds privileges, insists they wear state clothes on excursions to town, or transfers patients into or out of the program without the program director's permission or knowledge, the token economy is in serious trouble. Before the program begins, it is imperative that the director have the authority to make the necessary decisions for the program to operate effectively. It is helpful to have the token economy program as its own separate unit responsible directly to the hospital superintendent.

A token economy is a multidisciplinary program with built-in professional rivalries and petty jealousies. The director is faced with problems from the least expected sources and oftentimes for the most unbelievably trivial reasons. If the program is really going to run and run well, then every person with even the remotest connection to the program must be kept fully informed about everything that is going on within the program. At the very least, the hospital superintendent, the clinical director, and the director of nursing must be sent regular written reports in addition to verbal communications regarding all significant and not so significant happenings in the program. Minutes of all meetings must be kept and distributed to all staff members in the program. The director must be eternally vigilant to make sure everyone knows everything that is happening within the program.

STAFF TRAINING

Staff training never ends. First, some formal orientation using lectures, films, and informal group discussions is needed. Particularly helpful are role-playing sessions, where some staff members are asked to portray problem patients engaging in specific inappropriate behaviors, such as temper tantrums, noisy and messy eating, and "bugging" aides, while other members are asked to show how to deal with these behaviors. An initial two-week training session, including one-hour daily sessions covering the basic principles of behavior modification and specific goals of the program should be sufficient to give the staff an introduction to the treatment techniques. Topics to be covered in the training sessions might include:

1. What is Mental Illness?
2. Rights of Residents,
3. Principles of Behavior Modification,
4. Accountability,
5. Strengthening and Weakening Behaviors,
6. General Principles of a Token Economy,
7. Individual Behavioral Prescriptions, and
8. Mechanics of a Token Economy.

If the program is going to use volunteers, including college students and women from local clubs and service organizations, then it is important that they also receive the same training program as the hospital personnel; otherwise these well-meaning individuals will inevitably do more harm than good. After the initial two-week period, weekly training sessions, in which in-depth individual treatment plans are developed with all members of the treamtent team, including the ward aides, nurses, social worker, psychologist, and psychiatrist taking part are valuable in maintaining the morale of the staff members and in keeping them well-trained.

THE PUNCH CARD SYSTEM

To prevent poor economics from ruining a token program, the director must be ever alert to make sure tokens earned and tokens spent remain about the same for all patients (Winkler, 1973). All program directors know that the program can get out of balance very easily. Many patients beg, hoard, and steal tokens. Some patients use extortion to acquire tokens. Programs deal with these problems in many ways, such as by fining the culprits, or by devaluing tokens after a specific date to discourage hoarding, etc. These problems also make record keeping particularly difficult. One way to eliminate these problems and to run a token economy with increased control over earnings and spendings is to use a punch card system.

The punch card system is a method of awarding, collecting, and fining points through the use of cards which each patient carries with him at all times. These cards are used rather than actual tokens for several reasons:

1. Recording each token transaction in a ward logbook is eliminated because the interaction is recorded on the card.
2. The card is an accurate representation of the patient's activities at all times.
3. The staff has considerably less paperwork and therefore more time for interaction with the patients.
4. Begging, hoarding, and stealing of tokens are eliminated, resulting in much tighter controls over reinforcers.

Figure VIII-1 represents the punch card* used in the token economy program at Florida State Hospital. The card consists of three sections: tokens earned, tokens spent, and tokens fined.

The "Tokens Earned" section lists various activities that the patient may engage in to earn points, e.g. personal hygiene, cleaning on the ward, off-ward work, participating in occupational therapy (OT) and music therapy (MT), attending educational classes (Educ.), giving tours of the ward, serving as ward president or secretary, etc.; and the number of points to be paid for taking part in each activity. A list of appropriate personal hygiene requirements is posted on each token ward, along with the value of each activity, e.g. shower, two points; brush teeth, two points; shave, two points; comb hair, two points, etc. A list of ward cleaning tasks with the point values for each task is also posted on each ward and the task each patient chooses (or is assigned) is written on the card after the word "cleaning." The item, "Individual Earnings," represents the particular behaviors being worked on with each patient, i.e. the individual behavioral prescription. These prescriptions, written on the back of each patient's card and in each ward medical chart, include instruc-

---

* The punch card was designed by Ms. Susan LaFehr, Department of Psychology, Florida State Hospital, Chattahoochee, Florida.

TOKEN ACCOUNT CARD

1	2	3	4	5	5		Personal Hygiene	wk.	bal.	
5	6	7	8			TOKENS EARNED				
10	10	10	5	5	5		Cleaning	10	10	10
10	10	10	5	5	5			10	10	10
10	10	10	5	5	5		Off ward work 25	10	10	10
10	10	10	5	5	5		O.T. 15 M.T. 15	10	10	10
10	10	10	5	5	5		Educ. 25 Tour ldr. 5	10	10	10
10	10	10	5	5	5		Pres. or Sec. 25	10	10	10
							Individual Earnings	5	5	5
								5	5	5
							TOTAL EARNINGS			
10	10	10	5	5	5	TOKENS SPENT	Room Rent	D.S.C		
10	10	10	5	5	5		Meals 15			
10	10	10	5	5	5		Dayroom 15	10	10	10
5	5	5	5	5	5		Games, Crd, Rdo, TV 5	10	10	10
5	5	5	5	5	5		Ground Priv. 15 Ltd. 5	10	10	10
5	5	5	5	5	5		Town Priv. 15	10	10	10
5	5	5	5	5	5		Naps-sleeping 15	10	10	10
5	5	5	5	5	5		Social act. 5 Dance 15	10	10	10
5	5	5	5	5	5		Money 5 Talk staff 5	10	10	10
5	5	5	5	5	5		PRN Med. 10	10	10	10
5	5	5	5	5	5		Apt. with prof. 10	10	10	10
5	5	5	5	5	5		Beauty Shop 10	10	10	10
5	5	5	5	5	5		Ind. Therapy 15	10	10	10
							Individual Spending	5	5	5
								5	5	5
							TOTAL SPENT			
10	10	10	10	5	5	TOKENS FINED	Stealing 50			
10	10	10	10	5	5		Dest. of prop. 50			
10	10	10	10	5	5		Fighting 50			
10	10	10	10	5	5		Vulgar Lang. 25			
10	10	10	10	5	5		Not signing out 50			
10	10	10	10	5	5		Throw thg at pers. 25			
10	10	10	10	5	5		Smoking in bed 50			
10	10	10	10	5	5		In prob. area 25			
10	10	10	5	5	5		Creating Distb. 15			
10	10	10	5	5	5		Distb. aft. L.O. 10			
10	10	10	5	5	5		Lying-False Rpt. 15			
5	5	5	5	5	5		Bug. st. 5 Ing. Int. 5			
5	5	5	5	5	5		Litter.-Items/Box 5			
5	5	5	5	5	5		Throwing things 5			
5	5	5	5	5	5		Bottles on unit 5			
10	10	10	5	5	5		Late Return 25/hr.			
10	10	10	5	5	5		Not up on time 10-35			
10	10	10	5	5	5		Begging 25			
10	10	10	5	5	5		Unpaid radio 25			
10	10	10	5	5	5		Unpaid privilege 15			
10	10	10	5	5	5		Unpaid sleep 20			
10	10	10	5	5	5		Missing Therapy 10			
10	10	10	5	5	5		Missing med. call 25			
10	10	10	5	5	5		Missing 2nd meal 25			
10	10	10	5	5	5		Ref. job assig./wk.			
10	10	10	5	5	5		Bed area messy 5-25			
10	10	10	5	5	5		In chr. rm. w/o per. 15			
10	10	10	5	5	5		Tearing up card 25			
10	10	10	5	5	5		Loosing card 15			
10	10	10	5	5	5		Forgetting wk. cd. 25			
10	10	10	5	5	5		Loosing wk. card 25			
							Individual fining			
							TOTAL FINED			

FLORIDA STATE HOSPITAL
PSYCHOLOGY DEPARTMENT
TOKEN ECONOMY PROGRAM

Figure VIII-1.

tions to the ward aides and other staff members, e.g. "reward Mary two points each time she initiates a conversation," "reward Betsy two points each time she washes her own clothes," "ignore Williams when he talks to himself," "ignore Peter when he discusses his participation in Watergate or when he says he works for the FBI," etc. These represent individual behaviors being shaped or extinguished and differ from patient to patient. Usually, a maximum of two to three individual behaviors are included in the prescription at any one time and prescriptions are revised frequently.

The second section of the card is entitled "Tokens Spent." This section includes all privileges requiring points, including room rent, meals, use of dayroom, games, cards, renting a radio, watching television, grounds privileges, limited grounds privileges (for short visits etc.), town privileges, extra naps, dances and social activities, checking out money, meetings with staff members, PRN medication (aspirins etc.), appointments with professional personnel, appointments at the beauty shop, individual therapy with the psychologist, etc. Room rent varies from two points a night for large fifteen-bed rooms, to twenty-five points a night for private bedrooms. The item, "Individual Spending," includes any particular activity not covered in the other categories.

The third section is entitled "Tokens Fined" and lists inappropriate costly behaviors including stealing, destruction of property, fighting, vulgar language, not signing the ward logbook when leaving the ward, throwing things at persons, smoking in bed or in prohibited areas, creating a disturbance on or off the ward, disturbing the ward after lights out in the evening, lying, bugging staff (i.e. inappropriate behavior toward staff members), ignoring instructions from ward staff, littering, throwing things, and leaving soft drink bottles on the ward. Other costly behaviors include late return to the ward; not getting up on time; begging; using a radio or utilizing other privileges without paying; sleeping at inappropriate times; missing therapy, medicine call, or two meals in a row; refusing a weekly job assignment; not cleaning bed area; entering the chart room without permission; tearing or losing the card; or forgetting or losing one's assigned job time card. There is also a space for individual fining which is used for any other costly behaviors not covered. Although the card may make the economy look more like a fining than a reinforcing one, such is not the case, for in reality, many more behaviors are rewarded with points than are fined and staff members constantly try to keep fining at an absolute minimum.

All points earned, spent and fined during the day are punched in the columns on the left side of the card. The three columns on the right side of the card are used to punch out the current weekly bank balance (wk. bal.) on the top part of the card and the special spendings (from either the current weekly bank balance or from their savings account on the back of card) on the center part of the card. The letters D.S.C. stand for "drink stand card" and under the letters is written in the cost of this card (usually 200 points), which may be paid for out of the current weekly bank balance or the savings account.

All key staff members have their own individualized card punches. Each punch has a special die (e.g. including letters of the alphabet, symbols of hearts, diamonds, etc.), so that it can be determined which staff members punched the patients' cards. Ward aides are assigned four patients each and they have the primary responsibiilty for punching the cards of their patients each day.

The punches with the special dies prevent patients from buying their own punches and rewarding themselves with unearned points. These special punches can be ordered from several sources including McGill Metal Products Company, General Office and Factory, Marengo, Illinois 60152.

Each patient receives a new card daily, although it is also possible to make each card last a week by reducing the number of points paid, charged, and fined.

Each night the assigned staff member collects the cards and totals each one, subtracting the points spent and fined from the points earned. These data are first recorded on the back of the card along with any notes regarding unusual patient behaviors, and the amounts are also recorded on ward charts. The balance is tabulated and punched out on the weekly balance section of the new card (Figure VIII-2) the patient is to receive the next day. If spendings and finings exceeded earnings, the negative balance is subtracted from the already accumulated weekly

	Name		
	Date		

Bank		
Fine	WD	Bal.
Deposit		
Balance		

Bank

Fining or spending

Notes

Earned_____
Fined_____
Spent_____

Week Bal.	_____
Total earned	_____
Total spent	_____
Total fined	_____
Balance	_____
D.S. savings	_____
Deposit	_____
New Wk.Bal.	_____

Figure VIII-2.

balance, or if there is no balance, it is subtracted from the savings account. At the end of the week, the weekly balance is added to the patient's savings account.

Patients are expected to live off the front of the card, i.e. their daily expenses are paid with their daily earnings. The weekly balance is generally used only for special items and privileges, such as the weekly drink stand card, visits on the ward with relatives, long-distance phone calls, etc. Savings accounts are normally used only for certain important items or privileges, including purchase of expensive clothes from the hospital clothing store, special visits with relatives or friends off the hospital grounds, weekend passes, extended leaves of absence, etc. A running balance is kept on all patients so that the staff is immediately aware of any tendency toward a lopsided ward economy.

This punch card system, although perhaps sounding complicated, is really not difficult for ward aides and other staff members to learn. Since all ward personnel carry punches, point reinforcement for appropriate behaviors can be given quickly, along with immediate social reinforcement. Complete records are available on all patients, including points earned, spent, and fined; and what staff members are doing the reinforcing and how many points they are awarding or charging.

Hoarding is eliminated because patients are required to live off the front of their card, i.e. they meet their daily expenses with their daily earnings. Stealing is eliminated since each card has the patient's name written on it; and other than the card, which is worthless for anyone other than the one to whom it was issued, there is nothing of value to steal. When a puncher is stolen from a staff member, the special die symbol is declared worthless, so that any punches showing that symbol are without value. Extortion is eliminated because one patient cannot take punched holes from another, and the card itself is worthless to anyone other than the patient whose name is on it.

Many of the problems that arise within token programs can be reduced by stricter controls over administering the economy. A tighter economy, such as this punch card system, will help decrease unresponsiveness particularly with the use of many backup reinforcers, since the program requires that patients need to live off the front of the card, i.e. meet daily expenses with daily earnings.

Most staff and patients of the token economy program at Florida State Hospital report that they like the punch card system better than the previous system where plastic tokens were used. It seems to be easier on both staff and patients since staff members find they have more time to spend with patients on the ward, and patients no longer have to worry about losing their tokens or getting them stolen. With these tighter controls, more patients should be responsive to the program.

To date, one type of patient, the antisocial personality, has consistently been unaffected by the program. The token system at Florida State Hospital failed to change the unsocialized psychopathic behaviors of all four patients showing this personality pattern who went through the program. Apparently, the controls available at the hospital are not sufficient to enable staff members to effect any significant behavioral changes with these patients. The program has solved the problem of the psychopathic patient by refusing to admit them to the token economy wards. Alcoholics have also been unaffected by the program and probably require some more drastic behavior therapy approach, such as aversion therapy. Obsessive-compulsive patients with long histories of bizarre, ritualistic behaviors have made relatively few changes in their inappropriate behaviors through this program. Again, behavior therapy, using aversive conditioning, might help with these extremely difficult to treat patients.

COMMUNITY ADJUSTMENT

The ultimate goal of most token economy programs in mental institutions is to teach the patient the necessary skills to adjust outside of the institution. Unfortunately, there have been few studies examining the adjustment of former token economy patients in the community. Davison (1969, p. 278) stated the problem this way: "The overall evaluation of behavior modification in institutional settings was less than completely enthusiastic, primarily because of the failure of at least the operant approaches, thus far, to make an appreciable contribution to the goal of equipping adult mental hospital patients with the means to cope successfully in the outside world." Kazdin and Bootzin (1972, p. 360), after an extensive review of the token economy literature, concluded that "although token economies have been dramatically effective at changing behavior within the psychiatric hospital, there is little evidence that improvement is maintained outside the institution."

The major indices used to judge the success of token economies generally have included comparative discharge rates and recidivism rates. Comparing the discharge rate of a token economy program to that of other hospital programs that did not involve comparable therapeutic attention and the same general living conditions is perhaps more indicative of the value of administrative decisions and hard-working social workers than of therapeutic effectiveness. The reporting of comparative discharge rates is generally not very informative, since data (e.g. ages, hospitalization time, diagnoses, etc.) on patients released from other programs are rarely given. Information concerning recidivism rates is usually more helpful, but few studies have reported any long-term data (exceptions include Birky, et al., 1971; Foreyt, et al., 1975; Heap, et al., 1970; and Shean and Zeidberg, 1971). The most telling criticism of current token research in institutional settings is the almost complete lack of data on community adjustment of released patients.

In an effort to evaluate whether the program at Florida State Hospital does teach patients the skills to survive outside of the hospital, attempts are made to contact all released patients and they are asked to fill out a questionnaire dealing with their occupational adjustment, their use of community services (including local mental health centers, resources of the Divisions of Family Services, Vocational Rehabilitation, etc.), and their community adjustment. To date, sixty-one out of ninety-eight patients released over the past two years have been accounted for, either by returning the questionnaire (50 have returned the questionnaire) or by being readmitted to a hospital (11 have returned to a Florida hospital). With persistence and the help of counselors from Vocational Rehabilitation and Family Services, it is hoped several more will be cooperative and will complete the adjustment questionnaire. Preliminary data are encouraging. Several of the discharged patients, who had been hospitalized twenty to thirty years, have now been out of the hospital over two years and are living in apartments, apparently adjusting quite well to noninstitutional living. Several are working, either full- or part-time. Almost 80 percent of those responding to the questionnaire reported that their life is better since they left the hospital; about 20 percent reported their life is about the same as when they were in the hospital. None said their life is now worse than when they were in the hospital. Full details of this adjustment survey will be reported when it is completed (Hollingsworth, 1974) but these preliminary results suggest that this token economy does indeed equip at least some hospitalized psychiatric patients with the necessary skills to survive in the outside world.

SUMMARY

To maintain an effective token economy, tight controls over reinforcers are needed. The punch card system described is one way of tightening up an economy. If token economies are going to make a significant contribution to mental health programs by effectively teaching patients to cope outside of the institution, research data on patient adjustment are needed. Preliminary data on patients released from the token economy program at Florida State Hospital suggest that many patients do indeed adjust in the community.

REFERENCES

Birky, H. J.; Chambliss, J. E., and Wasden, R.: A comparison of residents discharged from a token economy and two traditional psychiatric programs. *Behav Ther, 2*:46, 1971.

Davison, G. C.: Appraisal of behavior modification techniques with adults in institutional settings. In Franks, C. M. (Ed.): *Behavior Therapy: Appraisal and Status.* New York, McGraw, 1969, pp. 220-278.

Foreyt, J. P.; Rockwood, C. E.; Davis, J. C.; Desvousges, W. H., and Hollingsworth, R.: Benefit-cost analysis of a token economy program. *Prof Psychol, 6*:26, 1975.

Heap, R. F.; Boblitt, W. E.; Moore, C. H., and Hord, J. E.: Behavior-milieu therapy with chronic neuropsychiatric patients. *J Abnorm Psychol,* 76:349, 1970.

Hollingsworth, R.: Follow-up Evaluation and Benefit-Cost Analysis of the Token Economy Program at Florida State Hospital. Master's thesis, in progress. Tallahassee, Florida State University, 1974.

Kazdin, A. E., and Bootzin, R. R.: The token economy: An evaluative review. *J Appl Behav Anal,* 5:343, 1972.

Shean, G. D., and Zeidberg, Z.: Token reinforcement therapy: A comparison of matched groups. *J Behav Ther Exp Psychiatry,* 2:95, 1971.

Winkler, R. C.: An experimental analysis of economic balance, savings and wages in a token economy. *Behav Ther,* 4:22, 1973.

AUTHOR INDEX

167

SUBJECT INDEX

171

DATE DUE

DEC 17 '79			
MY 15 '85			
GAYLORD			PRINTED IN U S A